TURIYA
MEDITATION

The State of Wakeful Sleep

Author: Ishan Kyan

Table of Contents

Chapter one

Introduction

Turiya is the context to which the three different states of consciousness are subjected and transcended. The states of consciousness are: arousing consciousness, dreaming, and dreamless sleekness. In the Hindu philosophy, Turiya is a simple awareness, chaturtha, paramahmsa.

The state above deep, dreamless sleep that activates the superconscious. Turiya is the fourth state of consciousness in which each man rests in Satchidananda ("eternal, eternally aware and ever fresh bliss"), Swami Sivananda says. The person has reached the final release from the ego- awareness and is united with the infinite spirit. Turiya refers both to Atman and to Brahman, the eternal self, who represent their divine union.

The single soul understands the three waking, dreaming and sleeping states in Turiya and transcends them. He moves beyond Brahman's gross presence in the matcrial world, Brahman's subtle dimension in the dream World, and deep sleep induces the infinite form. As a pure knowledge and joy, he knows its true nature. Therefore, in the outer world he is saved from desire, delusion and duality.

Turiya is not a State other than the bigger states, but as super consciousness penetrates all layers of reality. Ramana

Maharishi considers Turiya to be the only truth as the natural state which permeates the other Ones. The Mandukya Upanishad talks of Turiya as a pure consciousness that the mind can not explain, can not understand and can not be understood, but eventually realized as the one true self.

Because of its unique nature, Turiya can not be represented by any empirical science instrument. It has no unique or generic features, it's one without a second. Having less, no activity like formation, preservation, etc. can characterize it. Then, what is the meaning of the science of Turiya, it can be asked? Isn't it just like a horse's horns? Not at all. Not at all. When a person realizes that he or she is Turiya, he or she is released from finding external things. He is released from the false assumption of the incredible life and the false expectation.

Chapter Two

Turiya

Once you know what the desert's true nature is, you don't pursue the illusion of mirage and when you know how the fabric is really true, you are not afraid of the thought of the serpent being falsely superimposed on you. Ignorance, appetite, relation, aversion etc. destroy knowing oneself as Turiya. Identity of the self and Turiya are at the core of the Upanishads ' instruction. "This is Atman" (Ma. Up. 11), "Atman really is all this" (Chh. Up. Vxx. 2); Compare "That you are" (Chh. Up. Vi. Viii 7).

Turiya is not outside the three states.... It is as if the' complete discovery of the cord is distorted by the illusion of a snake. The seams are immediately known when ignorance disappears that veils the true nature of the seam. The knowledge of the cord is not the result of the snake's concept being distorted; the clothes have been around always. No other knowledge instrument is required when the illusory snake concept has been destructed to expose the string. Similarly, the destruction of such qualities as subjective awareness and objective knowledge shows the truth of Turiya, but the association with Turiya is not the direct result. For the realization of Turiya no other knowledge instrument is required. There is no longer a gap between the unknown, knowledge and the understood when Turiya is realized.

The scriptures and other knowledge tools are therefore designed to achieve cessation of the attributes mentioned in the text, which is concurrent with Turiya's achievement. (The different ways of knowledge used to justify Brahman's not duality actually form a part of the field of duality. The purpose of the ways in which duality is destroyed is to destroy the ways in which knowledge is destroyed; so, such factors of achievement as the proof and prover do not remain. (Swami Nikhilananda: The Upanishads Volume 2, p.237).

Turiya is not that which is conscious of the inner (subjective) world, nor that which is conscious of the outer (objective) world, nor that which is conscious of both, nor that which is a mass of consciousness. It is not simple consciousness nor is It unconsciousness. It is unperceived, unrelated, incomprehensible, inferable, unthinkable and indescribable. The essence of the Consciousness manifesting as the self in the three states, it is the cessation of all phenomena; It is all peace, all bliss and non—dual. This is what is known as the Fourth (Turiya). This is Atman and this has to be realized. (Mandukya Upanishads VII).

Our consciousness undertakes radical changes daily, with the flow of time as day and night expressed and removed. Nevertheless, we have failed to note these changes because of the usual existence and to accept them as part of our ordinary lives. Without looking at our everyday state of consciousness, we are struggling to discover the real mystery of our life.

Such regular changes in consciousness have been studied carefully and taught us how Yogic and Vedantic teaks can be used as portals to transcendence and cosmic consciousness.

There are interesting variations in our regular path to awareness. Our radical changes in consciousness through the waking, dreaming and deep sleep are most important. Even in a waking state, however, our consciousness changes by changing pattern in thinking, emotion and thought, action and contemplation, work and pleasure, connection and loneliness. The waking mind has its own periods of vision, creativity and imagination and sleeping or awake hours. Yet, more dream and deep sleep deviations occur.

In the visions, we lose our consciousness, our conscious mind and fall into a more creative state that is beyond our personal control. We don't know we're dreaming in the dream state. We do not remember our relationship with the waking state until we wake up from a dream. The mind is still dreaming, but with thoughts we do not control. The body and senses have been relaxing in the meantime. Our dreams can be chaotic, incoherent and unbalanced. Or they may offer a far beyond the waking stage elegance, wisdom, and inspiration.

During deep sleep the dream operation of the mind ceases and a more inwardly than dreamlike state is achieved. We don't have any ordinary deep sleeping or dreaming operation that we encounter as a state such as vacuum, darkness, void, or blankness. But the state of deep sleep is full of mysteries. The body and mind are refreshed in this state with subtle energies within, emerging out of the same darkness, darkness and inaction characteristic of deep sleep.

As modern science suggests, the brain as a whole is cleansed of toxins, blockages and harmful memory patterns. Our wake state knows nothing about deep sleep directly, only what a dream we can remember for a few minutes after we wake. We only get the feeling for deep sleep when we wake up to be well asleep in the morning. If we have troubled dreams or wake up at night, our rest is diminished by deep sleep.

The physical and psychological immunity without proper deep sleep brews strength and equilibrium leading to an inevitable breakdown of the body as a whole. What is the character of the deep sleep healing power? It is because we return to the center of our being, the central everlasting consciousness in us, not constrained by external corporal factors.

Our prana undertakes the same radical changes, together with our consciousness. Our senses and motor organs are put in a dream state while our breath deepens. Our breath is deeper in deep sleep and our prana is deeper. Our senses and motor organs in sleep are lost directly to us. We are vulnerable to environmental factors and therefore always have to sleep in a safe area. Our Prana as our consciousness is linked and harmonized with the hidden depths of the deep sleep, which appears to be a source of vital energy.

Vedic thought talks of the ultimate purpose of Selves-realization, a non-located awareness beyond the limits of ego, time, space and karma. This allows us to live beyond our minds in our true Self. It is our learning witness. This selves-knowing state is the secret center of our deep sleep, behind the darkness.

With regard to our day-to-day consciousness journey, we must understand that our true self is not just a waking state. It is the Self or consciousness behind all the 3 waking, dreaming and sleeping states. The inner core of consciousness is the fourth degree of unchangeable consciousness or continuous life. This in Vedantic philosophy, in particular in the Mandukya Upanishad, is called Turiya, which explicitly aims at teaching us the essence of the four states and how to go them.

Most of us consider our consciousness as a result of our mental activity during most of the waking state and dream. Consciousness is described in Vedic philosophy as consciousness beyond the mind and the body. Pure consciousness is not a kind of intellectual activity like thought, emotion, feeling or remembering. It is pure light, unlimited space. It is a state of being. It is not a conceptual substance, name, type or number, description or meaning. This inner consciousness. There is no external comparison, objective consistency or feel. The whole embodied world and all of its forms of matter, energy, life and mind are fundamentally beyond it. It is the Unseen, the Unknown Knower, as the Upanishads say.

The question arises, whether this suggested knowledge of the subconscious, which exists in dreams and deep sleep, really can be felt, or just supernatural imagination. Yogis believe that you can experience the condition straight and simply by practicing concentration, meditation, focused attention and sustained attention. In addition, we can easily increase mental strength and obtain an awareness of an infinite material inside us that is not constrained by time or space, birth or death by practicing Yoga, mantra and meditation. We can be forced into this ever awake spectator, not recognized by the transience of the outer world or the changing existence of the mind.

Chapter Three

Achieving Turiya

Each and every yoga secret is part of our everyday life concealed from our normal routines and activities– through days, months, seasons and years we see, hear, talk and breathe. Perhaps the biggest secrets are our endless knowledge and its various levels.

Consciousness, as the steady inner light behind the changes of external life, forms the basis of our creation. We naturally work through the instruments of body and mind. We are conscious beings. Our present presence in the set of knowledge in the worlds of time and space is but one of many lives. Knowledge enables us to feel and know ourselves, the inner truth out of which body and mind function. This is our very heart.

Yet we are largely unaware of the nature of our consciousness. We are so engaged in projecting our consciousness onto the outside world that we have profoundly forgotten its roots. Our challenging lives preclude us from understanding who we are, what (if anything) death survives and what our ultimate aim is. We are caught in our own corporeal image, which forgets our inner nature of light. Our transient lives mask our inner connection with the Eternal.

The consequence of that diversion is the fact that we are guided by external forces rather than internal awareness through confusion, desire and sorrow. We live on our tumultuous surface and often do not visit the calm oceans. In the dense material world, we seek outer satisfaction and ignore the hidden happiness in us.

Our lives are a great mystery and development of consciousness. This is our most important task to explore. We should be encouraged to research our own minds carefully, not only the outside world. We need to research the profound consequences of our daily activities by waking and sleeping to our self-knowledge. This self-examination has been around for long, as shown on the pages before us in the Indian spiritual tradition.

Aspirations are often thought of as fantasy, unreal and meaningless to everyday life. In reality, it has much more than we have been taught in the West to dream and sleep. Indian spiritual awareness brings a sense of aspirations that can help us live a wealthier and better conscious life.

Turiya or the Fourth State

Turiya or fourth state is the condition the human soul has to rest in during Sat-Chit-Ananda Svarupa or Nirvikalpa Samadhi, the higher Brahma consciousness. Three states, Jagrat, Svapna and Sushupti, exist for the Jiva in the mire of Samsara. Turiya is the disease that goes beyond all three of these countries. Therefore, the fourth or Turiya. Turiya is Brahman or Atman.

Brahman is the embodying of knowledge and happiness or Sat-Chit-Ananda Vigraha. He doesn't have a start or an end. He's the center of everything. He's for everyone a shelter, help and the Lord.

There are many languages, but one is the language of the heart and pictures. Cows have a lot of colour, but milk is one color.

Many become prophets, but the essential things are the same in their instruction. There are many schools of philosophy, but the goal is one. There are many views and worship practices, but one is the Brahman or Lord.

The Self, i.e. the Pipeelika Marga and the Vihanga Marga, are both routes through yoga. Like the ant slowly goes, the aspirant also moves slowly on the spiritual journey. To purify his hands, he practices Karma Yoga and then Upasana takes his mind steadily. Eventually he follows Jnana Yoga's path and eventually achieves life's purpose. This is Marga or the Ant-Way of Pipeelika. Just like the bird flies in the sky, so the first-class candidate practices Jnana Yoga concurrently and becomes acquainted with the self. That's the bird path or the Vihanga Marga.

You may equate man with an installation. It grows and thrives like a plant and dies at the end, but not entirely. The plant is also growing, thriving and eventually dying. The seed that grows a new plant is left behind. Man leaves behind the good and bad deeds of his life as he dies his karma. The physical body can die and rot, but his memories do not perish. To enjoy the fruits of these deeds, he must be born again. Every life can be the first because it is the result of previous deeds, not the last, because in the next life it must be expiated. Samsara would therefore be without beginning and end, or phenomenal life. But for a free wise man, there's no samsara who lives in his own Sat Chit Ananda Svarupa. There is not one of them. The Samskaras, which brings him into this world twice, are killed by man by acquiring knowledge of the Self and by being freed.

Have a thorough Upanishads analysis. No such inspiring and beneficial research can be found all over the world as Upanishads. Each mantra has powerful, original, sublime and emotional thoughts pregnant. They are the creations of the universal Rishis of India's highest awareness. They give the readers warmth, inner strength, harmony and courage. They instill faith in the hopeless, strength in the poor, harmony in the cheerful and serenity in the restless. The Vedanta system comes from the Upanishads that comprise the ancient wisdom of the ancient sages. A thorough examination of these majestic Upanishads demonstrates clearly how large the Rishis of Year had been in the Heart. The Western scientists are paying tribute to the Rishis and appreciating the beauty and originality of the Upanishads.

Argue not. Give up physical warfare, gymnastics and clubbing. When you get into arguments and disputes, you will not be anywhere. Have living faith or unshaking belief, the words of your Preceptor and the Shrutis, in the life of the sinful, all-pervading Brahmin or the Eternal. Learn the basic principles of Advaita Vedanta from your preceptor. The Advaita Vedantin accepts six Pramanas, but Shrutis is the last court of appeal. Srutis includes the inspired observations and insights of the wise. In the following, he also opens his Vedantic speeches. Srutis Bhagavati says, "Ekameva Advitiyam, Brahma, Sarvam Khalvidam, Brahma, etc.." Sruti Bhagavati says, most logic and reasoning are not necessary to understand and know the truth. The truth is quite clear. It can be done by simple meditation. Mind is only a finite resource. It is an autonomous and a regular professorship. It is not autonomous and self-luminous. You're going to be fooled. Intuition is unfailing or unfailing.

These well-qualified and well-equipped candidates will really profit from renouncing or Nivrittimarga. Many give up the world and in temporary zeal take Sannyasa. We do not proceed on the spiritual way, as without spiritual life there is no training and qualifications.

The one who sits by physically calming his mind, who does nothing, is the most active person in the world; whereas the other who runs here and there and always is really busy, does nothing significantly. You may think this is paradoxical. Very few can say that.

Husk is normal to rice and rust to copper, but through efforts it disappears! Evan so Ajnana which clings to the Jiva or individual soul can be caused by the uninterrupted Atmic inquiry to disappear. Kill Avidya. Kill Avidya. -you remain in your own self incomparably strong!

Don't confuse Tandri with Savikalpa Samadhi and Nirvikalpa's deep sleep. Turiya and Huma are ineffable glories. The magnificence can not be represented. If your body is warm, if your mind is clear if you are content, know that you are meditating. If your body is heavy, you know that you slept while meditating, if your mind is quiet.

Death comes from ignorance and lust. The deathless or eternal Atman is done with experience. By experience. Eternal life as well as death sleep in the body. Life is a spark or a blast of lightning. Time is but death's blowjob. Sleep at Atman. Sleep at Atman. You're going to achieve salvation. Go over time. Go over time. You are going to reach heaven.

Drop the Indriyas. Fall Indriyas. Think about it. Meditate. Live by yourself. Live by yourself. The whole being is taken to a kind of rapture or divine pleasure. You are going to feel the joy of Heaven. Great peace is going to encircle you. In the seas of paradise, you'll be lost. Each wish must melt all names and forms into nothingness. Just everywhere can you look at the Self. This glorious state can not be represented. You will see it yourself. You will. Just as a stupid man can not express the joy of eating the sugar-candy, so you can not communicate the satisfaction of Samadhi or the Supreme Self. This condition is finite in terms. This experience is not ideal for language. It's the ultimate silence term. It is an everlasting mind's absolute silence. Peace has passed all understanding. Turiya or the fourth state.

The Fourth State of Mind

Know you what the fourth state is? The human mind is a magnificent and powerful piece of complex machinery that can calculate much more rapidly and much more accurately than a supercomputer. In particular, in order to properly understand the consciousness (Turiya) in particular the various states of mind that we encounter should be understood.

There are majorly two parts of the human mind: Subconscious Mind

Conscious Mind

Conscious mind is the analytical and essential part of our brain which at any time controls our awareness or consciousness. It's the final result of our daily decisions, actions or reactions. It controls our strength of will, long-term memory, logical thought and critical thought. At present, the mind of consciousness is actually the consciousness. You know something on the outside and you know other mental functions on the inside.

Subconscious Mind is the' deeper' part of the mind which processes thousands of events at any given time and stores all we experienced at different levels in our lives. It's kind of an' auto pilot' and doesn't even know what happened to us. It is similar to a computer hard drive which saves information accessed through the other parts of the computer. This controls our convictions, feelings, behaviors, ideals, defensive responses, creativity, insight and some of the longer-lasting memory that is stored in our brains. (many scholars mention the unconscious mind that also typically regulates the automatic processes of the physical body).

The mind operates at four dominant brainwave states or frequencies.

Digital EEG Machine

These various states are classified at any point in time according to the intensity of the prevailing brainwave signals. This velocity is measured in' Hertz' and the figures obtained via an electrical cardiograph machine (EEG).

Beta: Here is where our mind usually works every day. We are fully aware of everything around us in such a state and we have little emphasis. Typically, only one side of our brain works at this stage. The higher cycles of beta frequency are usually equated with tension, anxiety and "over thinking" as the mind misdirects, or responds negatively to, a given situation. Beta can be described in the brainwave cycles of 15 to 40 Hz (cycle per second) High brainwave beta also equates to high blood pressure, increased respiratory rate, increased blood flow, release of cortisone and glucose. Speaking generally, if you are concerned about your health, you don't want to have the high beta condition too often. (Some strategies to ensure this is not mentioned below).

Alpha: A mild relaxing state or a faint daydream. If you are driving a car, and cruising around, or if you get stuck in a good book and somehow lose track of what is taking place around you, the Alpha activity can be an example. Meditation is usually done to oscillate Alpha frequency of your brain waves. In cycles between 9Hz and 14Hz, the brain then works. Alpha is generally regarded as a combination of partial consciousness and partial subconscious predominance. If your brain is in alpha frequency it is helpful to absorb information, and it is considered extremely desirable for successful studying and concentrating. The left side of the brain is used by alpha for processing.

Theta: A profound rest where most of the conscious spirit is "displaced" and the subconscious spirit is allowed to thrive and walk through its own path. This is usually characterized by sleep, dreaming, very deep relaxation and is where the majority of hypnotizers want their guests. THETA exhibits a 5-Hz to 8-Hz brainwave interval. This is where thoughts, visualizations and suggestions reach the subconscious mind and we become consciously unaware of what's happening around us.

Delta: Extremely deep sleep / relaxation with a fully functioning subconscious mind. Delta is encountered in the deepest of the sleep and it is interesting because it has been shown that at this stage the physical body begins to regenerate and heal. You can be in an advanced state of meditation in waking delta. This state is linked to the experiences of kundalini. Deep brainwaves at 1Hz-4Hz are typified for delta. It is worth noting that a high-quality hypnotist who is able to take a client to the Delta State will carry out the practice by using hypnosis as a replacement for anesthesia during various medical operations.

Transitioning Between the Different States

Since the human mind naturally changes according to the environment, the scenario, the people or events of the person between various states of mind. You may activate the brain artificially at different levels. An extreme example is that we sometimes go to coma when we are involved in a serious accident or injury. This is the way the mind reacts to an emergency and reaches the deepest realms of the Delta immediately for increased physical healing, wound safety and mental healing. This is an excellent example of the natural reaction of the brain when it reduces brainwave activity in order to protect it instinctually.

In both constructive and sometimes beneficial reasons, we can deliberately cause a shift in our mental state. Stage hypnotists also invite theta for entertainment purposes to a sudden change in the strength of the brain wave by a quick hypnotic induction. Although it is amusing for most people and shows the power of hypnosis, it has only a chuckle that is not really a good purpose. There are several examples of reckless use of these mass manipulation techniques and these are clearly a disastrous use of something so effective for positive change.

There are many ways to invoke an individual artificially in different states of brainwave frequency. These include hypnosis, meditation, music and audio, massages, food, alcohol, exercise, Pilates, video games, tv, driving, reading etc. In discovering the best way to reduce your mind to Alpha, Theta and Delta, you will create multiple positive emotional, mental and physical advantages. Hypnosis, for example, is perfect to expose you to theta, and then make responsible use of direct advice, which your unconscious mind better accepts, to create positive and enduring changes in your mind and body.

Meditation is also useful to create a light Alpha state in which information and self-suggestions can be processed effectively to help the emotions and feelings change. Music and sound, such as binaural beats, white sound, theta rhythm, nature recordings, etc., can help you to resolve insomnia and sleep better, carry out self-meditation, self-hypnosis, and achieve profound relaxation in the alpha, theta, and, often, the delta. Deep relaxation on a daily basis has proved useful to the mind and body! This promotes clarity of thought, focus, better health and enhanced well-being of mind, physical and emotions.

The fourth mental condition is similar to the realization of God or the super consciousness. This is mentioned in a great ancient philosophical text.

Chapter Four

The Upanishad

The Upanishads are ancient Sanskrit teaching texts and Hindu beliefs, mostly followed by religious traditions such as Buddhism and Jainism. It is one of the oldest writings in the Hindu, the Vedas, which deal with meditation, philosophy and spiritual knowledge; other parts of the Vedas deal with mantras, blessings, rituals, ceremonies and sacrifices Of ancient times the Upanishads played an important part in the development of spiritual ideas in one of the main literatures in the history of Indian religions and culture.. The Upanishads alone are widely recognized of all Vedic literature and their main concepts are at the spiritual heart of Hinduism.

Currently the Upanishads are called Vedanta. The concept of Vedanta as "last chapters, parts of the Veda" and as "Subject, the highest aim of the Veda." These are the central ideas in all Upanishads and the center of the philosophy of Brahman (the last reality) and Tetman (the mind, the self). They are their thematic matter. Two prominent monistic schools of Hinduism are established along with the Bhagavad Gita and the Brahmasutra, the mukhya Upanishads (known collectively as Prasthanatrayi).

There are more than 200 Upanishads known, about the first dozen are the oldest and most significant, and the main

Upanishads (mukhya). The mukhya Upanishads are found mostly in the latter part of the Brahmanas and Aranyakas and have been recalled and transmitted orally for centuries by each generation. The early Upanishads were pre-Common Period, of which five were possibly pre-Buddhist (6th century BC), ranging from 322 to 185 BC into Maurya. Of the others, 95 Upanishads are part of the canon of Muktika from the last century to about the fifteenth century A.C. New Upanishads were still written in the early modern and modern period after 108 in the Muktika canon but were mostly concerned with subjects not related to the Vedas.

In the early 19th century they have begun to attract attention from a west audience with the Upanishads ' translation. The Upanishads influenced Arthur Schopenhauer profoundly, calling it "the development of the highest human knowledge." The philosophical aspects of the Upanisads and major Western thinkers were discussed in the modern era.

The term Upani Tad in Sanskrit (from up to "up" and "neither" to "sit") means that the student is sitting next to the teacher and gaining spiritual knowledge. Many examples of the dictionary include "esoteric idea" and "secret guidance." Monier-Williams ' Sanskrit Notes: "The Upanishad means to show the supreme spirit's knowledge and put a stop to ignorance."

Over 200 Upanishads are known, of which one, the Muktika Upanishad, was built up in 1656 and includes a list of 108 Canonical Upanishads. These were further split into Upanishad, aligned with shakti, sannyas, Shaivism (the god Shiva), yoga and sāmānya (general and sometimes referred to as Sāmānya-Vedanta), and Shaivism (the god Vishnua). These are also divided into the Shaktish.

Some Upanishads are called "sectarian" because they pose their ideas by a particular god or goddess of a different Hindu tradition, like Vishnu, Shiva, Shakti or a combination of those, like the Upanishad of Skanda. Such traditions tried to connect their Vedic texts, thus affirming the Upanishad, Čruti, in their language. Much of these secular Upanishads, for instance the Rudrahridaya Upanishad and the Mahanarayana Upanishad, contend that all the Hindu gods and goddesses are the same, that they are an all-embracing feature and manifestation of Brahman.

Mukhya Upanishads

It is possible to split the Mukhya Upanishads into sections. Brhadaranyaka and Chandogya, the oldest, are among the early ages.

Early in the middle of the 1th century BCE, the Aitareya, Kau Fastidieni and Taittiriya Upanishads date from around the 4th to 1st centuries BCE, approximately corresponding with earliest Sanskrit epics. There is a chronology suggesting that after the 5th century BC Aitareya, Taittiriya, Kausitaki, Mundaka, Prasna, Katha Upanishads had an influence on the Buddha; another suggestion challenges the assumption and dates it regardless of the date of birth of buddha. Following these major Upanishads, Kena, Mandukya and Isa Upanishads are generally placed, but these are other scholars. There is little knowledge of the writers except those mentioned in the texts, such as Yajnavalkayva and Uddalaka. Occasionally, a number of women are also present, such as Gargi and Maitreyi, Yajnavalkayva's aunt.

Each of the major Upanishads may be affiliated with one of the four Vedas (shakhas) exegesis colleges. Several Shakhas, of which only a few remain, are said to exist. The modern Upanishads often have little connection to the Vedic corpus and have not been mentioned or commented upon by any great Vedanta philosopher: their language varies from that of the classical Upanishads, being less descriptive and more formalized. As a result, they are not difficult for the average reader

to understand.

New Upanishads

The Upanishads have not been classified as recent ones, but have been discovered and written beyond the Muktika anthology of 108 Upanishads. In 1908, for example, Friedrich Schraders, who attributed it to the first Upanishad prose, revealed four previously unknown Upanishads in newly found manuscripts called Bashkala, Chhagaleya, Arsheya and Saunaka. The text of three of them was incomplete and incomplete, probably poorly preserved or corrupted, namely the Chhagaleya, Arsheya and Saunaka.

Ancient Upanishads have long been respected for Hindu tradition and writers of different sectarian texts have sought, by calling their texts Upanishads, to benefit from this reputation. Such hundreds of "new Upanishads" cover various topics from biology to rejection of sectarian theory. It consisted of the early modern era (~1600 CE) from the last decades of the first millennium BC. Although more than two dozen minor Upanishads date back to the previous 3.00 CE, many of these new texts with the title "Upanishad" came into being during the first half of the 2nd millennium CE. For example, the main Shakta Upanishads specifically discuss doctrinal and interpretative differences between the two main Tantric sects of a major shakticism known as Shri Vidya upasana. The many lists available for the authentic Shakta Upani Godads differ, representing the sect of their compilers, to prevent them from providing proof that they "locate" in the tantric tradition. The content of tantric texts weakens even their status as a Upani lifestyle. Sectarian texts like these are not considered shruti and thus the authority of the modern Upanishads is not recognized as a scripture in Hinduism.

The four Vedas– Rigvida, Samaveda, Yajurveda (the two main versions or Yajurveda Samhitas– are Shukla Yajurveda, Krishna Yajurveda, and Atharvaveda) all are related to Upanishads. During the modern era, the ancient Upanishads that were rooted in texts in the Vedas were removed from the Vedic layers of Brahman and Aranyaka, compiled into distinct texts and collected in Upanishads anthology. The lists are related to one of the four Upanishads and are many of them, and in all of India these lists are inconsistent with the Upanishads and the manner in which the newer Upanishads are supposedly assigned to the old Vedas. The list collected in South India was made the most popular by the 19th century based on Muktika Upanishad, and was written in Telugu. The 52 Upanishads were most famous in northern India.

The list of Muktika Upanishads contains 108 Upanishads the first thirteen as Mukhiyas, twenty like Sāmānya Vedanta, ten like Sannyasa, fourteen like Vaishnava, twelve as Shaiva and eight as Shakta. Two as Yoga. The following table shows 108 Upanishads recorded in the Muktika. The most important and outstanding mukhya Upanishads are.

A plurality of worldviews characterized the Upanishadic era. While some Upanishads are considered to be' monitory,' others are dualist, including the Katha Upanishad. In comparison to the non-dualistic Upanishads at the base of its Vedanta school, Maitri is one of the Upanishads who tend toward dualism that form the classical Samkhya and the Yoga School of Hinduism. We have a variety of ideas.

The Upanishads have inspired Indian thought as well as faith and life since their conception, says Sarvepalli Radhakrishnan. Only because they were discovered (Shruti) are respected by the Upanishads, but because they provide compelling philosophical ideas. The Upanishads are treaties of Brahmanism that is facts of the absolute hidden truth. "It is a strictly personal effort to reach the facts" their analysis of philosophy presumes. Word is a road to liberation in the Upanishads, Radhakrishnan says, and pursuit of knowledge by way of life is the philosophy.

The Upanishads includes metaphysical theory sections which were at the heart of Indian traditions. Chandogya Upanishad, for instance, contains one of Ahimsa's (non-violence) earliest known concepts of ethics. In the most ancient Upanisads and a large number of later Upanishads are also discussion of other ethical principles such as Damah (temperance) and self-restraint, Satya (truthfulness), Dāna (charity). The Brhadaranyaka Upanishad, the oldest Upanishad is stated likewise in the Karma doctrine.

Maitri Upanishad

In the oldest Upanishads the opposition to the practice is not explicit. At times, the Upanishads expand the task of the Aranyaka with a ritual allegorical and philosophical significance. The Brihadaranyaka, for instance, interprets horse sacrifice practice or allegorical Ashvamedha. It states that by sacrificing a horse, the over-lordship of the world can be acquired. Then it is said that only through the renunciation of the universe conceived as a horse can spiritual autonomy be achieved.

Similarly, the Vedic gods like Agni, Aditya, Indra, Rudra, Visnu, Brahma and others are in the Upanishads equaled with the ultimate, eternal and infinite Braham-Atman, God is identical with the self and is proclaimed to be everywhere in every human being and in every living creature. Ekam Eva Vitiyam or "one and the other and without a second" in Upanishads is the one reality or Ekam Sat of the Vedas. In the Upanishad, Brahman-Atman and self-realization develop as the road to the moksha (free life and freedom).

The thinkers of Upanishadic texts can, according to Jayatilleke, be divided into two classes. One community, which included early Upanishads and some mid- to late Upanishads, was made up of metaphysicians who used rational arguments to empirical experience to formulate their philosophical assumptions and speculations. The second group consists of many Upanishads, who professed theories based on yoga and personal experience. Yoga theory & practice is "not completely absent in the Early Upanishads," adds Jayatilleke. In these Upanishadic theories theory evolved within contrast with Buddhism, as a soul (Atman) is assumed to be the Upanishadic inquiry, while a Buddhist believes that there is no soul, states Jayatilleke.

Brahman and Atman

In the Upanishads Brahman and Atman are two ideals of prime importance. The Brahman is the ultimate reality and the Atman is the spirit. Brahman is the material explanation for what happens, accurate, formal and final. It is the all-encompassing, sexless, eternal, eternal truth and happiness, but the root of all transformation. Brahman, "is the eternal, manifested and non-manifest root, substance, center and destiny of all creation, the shapeless infinite substratum, from which the universe formed."

"The creative concept that is known all over the World is Brahman in Hinduism," Paul Deussen says.".

The word Atman means a person's inner self, the souls, the divine spirits and every living thing, including animals and trees. In all Upanishads, the main idea is the Tetman, and its thematic focus is "Know your life." These texts say that not the body, the mind, or the ego, but Atman– "soul," or "self"– is the inner core of every person. Atman is the spiritual essence of every person, its very essence. She's young, old. Athman is what you are at the lowest level of your life.

Atman is the main topic of the Upanishads, but two different themes are expressed. The two are rather divergent. Younger Upanishads state Brahman (the Highest Truth, Universal Concept, Being-Consciousness-Bliss) is the same as Atman, while former Brahman state Upanishads, Atman, but not the same. These somewhat conflicting ideas had been synthesized and merged by Brahmasutra from Badarayana (100 BCE). The Brahman sutras render Atman and Brahman both distinct and non-different, according to Nakamura, a view that was later called bhedabheda. Koller says that Brahman sutras claim that Atman and Brahman are different on some levels, particularly during ignorance, but that Atman and Brahman are identical and non-different on the deepest level and in the state of self-realization. This ancient debate has developed into several dual and non- dual Hindu theories.

Reality and Maya

According to Mahadevan, the Upanishads present two different types of the non-dual Brahman- Atman. The one wherein the non-dual Brahman-Atman is the universe's all-inclusive field, and the other where empirical, evolving truth appears (Maya).

The Upanishads describe the world and human experience as an interplay of Purusha (the universal, unchanging concepts of awareness) and Prak litti. The first is a tribune, the latter as a tribune, and Maya. The Upanishads describe Atman as "true knowledge" (Vidya) and Mayan knowledge as "not true knowledge" (Avidya and Nescience, lack of consciousness, lack of genuine knowledge).

"The term Maya was translated as' illusion' in the Upanishads, but then it does not include natural illusion," explains Hendrick Vroom. Myth' here doesn't mean that the world is not possible and is simply a human imagination construct. "To suggest, according to the Wendy Doniger" that the universe is an illusion (māyā) is not to say that the world is not possible; it is to say instead, that it is not what it seems, that it is something that is constantly being done. It means to be a reality, but a reality that we live through is deceptive in its true nature "Māyā does not just confuse people about what they claim to know; he limits their understanding more fundamentally.

Māyā is described in the Upanishads as the changing reality and he coexists with Brahman, the hidden true truth. Maya is an important idea for Upanishads, because the texts say it's Maya, which darken, confuses and distracts a person, in the human pursuit of happy and freeing self-knowledge.

Together with the Bhagavad Gita and the Brahmasutras, the Upanishads are one of the three principal origins of all Vedanta schools. The Upanishads have based their various interpretations on the variety of philosophical teachings. Vedanta schools strive to answer questions about atman and Brahman's relationship and about Brahman's relationship with the world. The Vedanta Schools are named after their friendship with Brahman:

There is no distinction, Advaita Vedanta says.

The jīvātman is a of Brahman, according to Vishishtadvaita, and is therefore related, but not identical.

All human souls (Jīvātmans) and matter, according to Dvaita, are immortal and separate beings.

Other schools in Vedanta include Dvaitadvaita of Nimbarka, Suddhadvaita of Vallabha and Bhedabheda of Chaitanya. The philosopher Adi Sankara wrote on 11 Upanishads of mukhya.

Advaita Vedanta

Advaita means non-duality literally and is a monistic theory of thought. This addresses Brahman and Atman's non-dual life. Advaita is the most influential sub-school of Hindu philosophy in the Vedanta School. In reflecting on the Upanishad comments, Gaudapada became the first person to reveal the fundamental principle of Advaita philosophy. Shankara (8th century CE), the Advaita ideas of Gaudapada, have been further developed. King declares that Mā Samukya Kārika, Gaudapadas principal work, is infused with Buddhism's philosophical terminology. King also notes that Shankara's writings are distinctly different from the Brahmasutra, and many of Shankara's ideas contradict those of the Upanishads. Radhakrishnan, on the other hand, indicates that Shankara's view about Advaita was straightforward production by the Upanishads and Brahmasutra.

In the discussions of the philosophy of the Advaita Vedanta, Shankara referred to the early Upanishads to explain the major difference between Hinduism and Buddhism, arguing that the Hindu is Atman (Soul, Self).

The Upanishads contain four sentences, Mahāvākyas, which Shankara used to describe Atman's and Brahman's identity as scriptural truth:

"Prajñānam brahma" – Aitareya Upanishad - "Consciousness is Brahman"

"Aham brahmāsmi" – Brihadaranyaka Upanishad - "I am Brahman" "Tat tvam asi" – Chandogya Upanishad - "That Thou art"

"Ayamātmā brahma" – Mandukya Upanishad - "This Atman is Brahman"

While the Upanishads are supported by many different philosophical views, commentators have usually followed Adi Shankara in seeing idealist monism as the dominant force.

Vishishtadvaita

Vedanta is the second school to be established by Sri Ramanuja (CE 1017–1137) by Vishishtadvaita. Adi Shankara and Advaita School were disagreed by Sri Ramanuja. Visistadvaita is a philosophy of synthesis that bridges the monistic Vedanta Advaita and theistic Dvaita systems. Sri Ramanuja also quotes the Upanishads and says the base of the Upanishads is Vishishtadvaita.

The study of the Upanishad by Sri Ramanuja's Vishishtadvaita is a trained monism. Sri Ramanuja interprets Upanishadic literature in order to teach theory of body mind, "notes Jeaneane Fowler– professor of philosophy and religious studies, who has Brahman as his soul, his inner power, his immortality. The Upanishads are the same qualities as the Brahman according to the Vishishtadvaita School but are distinct in quantity.

The Upanishads are interpreted at Vishishtadvaita School in order to teach an Ishwar (vishnu), who is the seat of all good qualities, with all the empirically conceived universe, as the body of God that resides in all life. The school encourages a commitment to godliness and a daily recollecting of personal god's beauty and love. It brings you eventually to the essence of Brahman abstract. Through Sri Ramanuja's interpretation, "The Brahman in Upanishads is a living reality," Fowler says, "the atman of all life and beings.".

Dvaita

Madhvacharya (1199–1278 CE) founded the third school in Vedanta, the Dvaita school. The presentation of Upanishads was considered to be profoundly theistic philosophic. Compared to Adi Shankara's arguments for Advaita and Sri Ramanuja for Vishishtadvaita, Madhvacharya says his theistic Dvaita Vedanta is based on Upanishads.

Fowler states: "The Upanishads who speak of the soul like Brahman speak of resemblance and not individuality," according to the school of Dvaita. Madhvacharya interprets Upanishadic lessons of oneself as "entering Brahman," just like a drop in the ocean. It implies duality and dependency for the Dvaita school, in which Brahman and Atman are different realities. Brahman is a separate, autonomous, supreme Upanishad reality. According to Madhvacharya, atman only resembles the Brahman in a minimal, less dependent way.

Sri Ramanuja Vishishtadvaita and Shankara's Advaita school are both non-dual schools of Vedanta; both are premised on the belief that all souls will be able to hope and reach a state of happy liberation.

The Mandukya Upanishad

The Upanishad was named after the sage Mandukya who taught the most exalted, including waking, dreaming, profound sleep and the fourth, Turiya. The third and fourth states are marked by the enigmatic syllable Om. The Upanishad also takes great care that Turiya is not a country, because this would characterize it. We will start with that understanding.

The Upanishad seems to be the shortest verse of just 12. Besides its implicit philosophy, Gaudapada's commentary, entitled Karika, made it renowned. In the sixth century A.D. Gaudapada existed. And it's said to be a mentor, or Govindapada's teacher who has been Shankaracharya's most famous tutor. While Advaita's philosophy or non-dualism is really the message of Upanishads, Shankaran's school has an elaborate exposure and its systematization.

The seven limbs are also the "cosmic body" called "vaisvanara" rather than the human body. They are stated in verse V.18.2 of the Chandogya Upanishad, which we are discussing later on. "The heavens are his hands, the sole of his eyes, the air is also his breath, the fire of his heart, the water his belly, the earth his feet, and the body room" is a translation from that Chandogya verse. These are the seven limbs that are defined in the Mandukya Upanishad's opening verse and clearly include the manifest universe. The "mouths" of nineteen include the 5 sensory bodies, the 5 action bodies (to walk, to speak, to eject, to procreate and to handle), the five pranas, the mind, the intellect, the ego sense and thought (citta).

The Upanishad goes on. "The second is the dream state, cerebral internally, with its seven limbs and nineteen mouths as well. The verse informs us that in the inner dream world there are parallels to all we find on our outside. In this state one encounters the implicit sensations of the mind." What we are experiencing in the waking state, we do have dream conditions but clearly not the same environment.

"Deep sleep or sleep without dream (prajna) is the third stage. When the day's night's darkness and the external world seem to vanish, the unconscious curtain includes thought and understanding also in sleeplessness, and the mental's subtle thoughts seem to disappear. It's a mass of consciousness, it's laughing, its face is imagined. In this case, the person is said to be happy because there is no tension or conflict. Prajna rules over everything, understands everything and is the inner master. It is the source and purpose of everyone. The fourth, turiya, is neither cognitive, nor internal externally, but cognitive in both directions. It is not a mass of cognition, not of a cognitive one, not of a cognitive one, not of a visible, incapable of being spoken about, inconspicuous, without any distinctive characteristic, unthinkable, unnamable, the nature of the one-elf knowledge, the friendly one, the benevolent one, the non-dual one. This is the blackbird. This must be done.

Here we see a word that shows the disorder beyond deep sleep for the first time. The mechanisms of waking and dreaming are causal and effectual. Prajna or the state of deep sleep is the only trigger. The ultimate thing, turiya, is beyond reason. Gaudapada writes in his Karika, "Prajna or the state of deep sleep knows no other things. The real or the imagined doesn't know it. They know nothing. They know nothing. But Turiya, fourth, knew it all and always knew it." We are completely unconscious in prajna state. In Turiya, you are not aware and unaware. You are' super viewed.' There is one thing in common with Prajna and Turiya. Both do not have a fantastic world vision. Prajna is sleeping though because he is ignorant, while Turiya is free from ignorance.

Upanishad continues, "Atman symbolized with omkara, which has four parts, having defined these 3 States and turiya, the" power "underlying them all and transcending them as well. The akara, or Om's sound, is the wake power and is the source of apti, which means" to get "and adimatva, and which means" to get first. "Everyone who knows this gets every urge and is the best of everything. Om's Ukara or U sound is the dream state, the root of the words utkarsa that mean' exaltation' and' intermediateness' is from ubhayatva. Who understands this, exemplifies and matches this concept in the strength of interpretation and consistency of knowledge? No one is born ignorant of Brahman is in his lineage,"

That needs to be explained. The waking state occupies the demonstrated world. There is no wish we can not satisfy if we truly understand the nature of this universe. Anyone absolutely understands this world is "the greatest of all." The first part of these verses is therefore plain. The second section is more profound. It includes dream state awareness. As stated in previous verse, in waking and dreaming states the realm of cause and effect is found. Modern psychoanalysis made a major attempt in an evaluation of dream state to comprehend behavior. The works of Carl Gustav Jung point to the "collective unconsciousness" where, whether we know this or not, archetypal images have a powerful influence over us. Therefore, in order to understand the waking state, the dream world must also be understood and that means "continuity of experience." Anyone who understands both of these is the same. The' lineage' in the verse is the series of students who learn from such a person. This legacy has a deeper philosophical dimension as none of these two consciousness systems can fully explain the nature of life.

The Upanishad states that' Prajna' is the state of deep sleep and is represented as makara or Om's m tone. This comes from the root mi, which means "to weigh" or "to combine." Anyone who understands all of this calculates, merges it into themselves. The fourth, turiya, is the silence of Om, the amatra which has no elements of which the universe is decided, fine, not double. So, Om is the atman syllable. Anyone who understands this knows Brahman.

Gaudapada's Karika is important to make the Mandukya Upanishad's initial systematic statement and at the same time to create the basis for advaita as instructed by Shankara. The Karika is well known for its example of "snake and chain." Gaudapada says that just as we recognize that dream image is simply our imagination, when we "wake" the consciousness of Brahman, we recognize that this world is simply our mental projection. "You see a cloth, at a dark place," writes Gaudapada, "but you don't know if you see a cloth. You're going to see a snake, a water pump, or something like that. These are all misunderstandings. There's just a cloth, you have the illusion that the fabric is a snake. "There's a great many other mirages because of this illusion. The snake does not live without the chain. The relationship between the world we see and Brahman is therefore exactly the same relationship between snake and rope. Likewise, the universe has no life apart from Brahman.' The distinction between all three countries and turiya is as is the disparity between the Waking and the Dream worlds.

The Taittiriya Upanishad

The Upanishad of Taittiriya is often referred to as the calling address because a list of ethical principles for life is given to the leaving students. It has also been well-known for its 5 layers, namely, food, breath, soul, soul, and happiness, or koshas of the human being. A "calculus of happiness" to the last Brahman is also delineated.

The Upanishad starts with a prayer for the teacher as well as for the taught person. One can see the tension on pronunciation from the second verse in those ancient times. "We are expounding pronunciation, letters, sounds, pitch, number, intensity or tension, joint and mixture. These are the pronunciation laws. It's a mix of this universe. The best variations are here. The earth is the first type. The latter form is heaven. The ether is the bond and the air are the connection."

Speech is the way the teacher communicates with the taught person. Therefore, voice, intonation and emphasis and variations of words are extremely important for a true meaning. Language is, in essence, the awareness of words combined, which in effect are sounds combinations. The combination description is therefore established for further analysis. The wise man explains how this idea is mirrored around us in the universe. The world starts because it is not distinct from the heavens but rather connected to the planet in space. As already pointed out, Brahman's teaching is the core of the Upanishad. Although it is beyond your imagination, you should extend your understanding of yourself and the entire world to grasp it.

"Now, knowledge is its relation, and the knowledge is the link," continues the sage, "the teacher is the prior form, the student is the latter form." In this verse the sage transmits to the student a celestial image in the light of teaching. It's a part of the universal cycle, not an isolated event. This dimension of meaning we must be conscious of.

Then there are verses that gave the Upanishad its subtitle as a' Call Address.' "Practice virtue," the sage instructs, "does not stop learning and teaching. Do not stop studying and teaching, practicing truth. Do not refrain from learning and teaching abstinence (tapas). Do not stop studying and teaching. Practice self-control. Practice tranquility, do not stop studying and teaching." Such verses are reverberative in the message Svadhyaya pravacane ca and imply "do not stop studying and teaching.". The famous Socrates statement: "Unexamined life is not worth living" provides a faint echo of this. We should always question ourselves, the world around us, and always keep from knowing. At the same time, we must remember that the transmission of information is part of a linking organic connection and that we must not avoid transmitting the legacy of knowing to future generations.

While explaining the importance of education, the sage advised his students not to neglect social duties: "Matr devo Bhava, pitr devo bhava, acarya devo Bhava, an antithi devo bhava." "Your mother should be a god to you, your father would be a god for you, your teacher would be a god to you and your guest a God to you." We always forget that the Mother is for our only protection, our only protector, our first teacher, for at least the formative years. After that, the dad comes, the coach, the visitor instead. Here is also the seed of a teaching which comes in the form of karma yoga in the Bhagavad Gita later whose key message is the science of practice.

The sage instructs his students very humbly, "There is good behavior. Don't copy our shortcomings. Just emulate in our practices what's great! Giving with faith, humility and compassion whatever you giving. If any concerns or suspicions about any matter arise, seek the advice of the learned and the wise and act accordingly after reflection. So, we should not be reckless about our behavior. This is the lesson. "If there is a question, we can consult the wise, (not the other, as Plato says), and then act accordingly. This is also said that the four' R's' are basic education. We need to teach reflection in while also teaching reading, writing and arithmetic. We may conclude from this passage that the ancients have been taught.

The sage now continues his comprehensive teaching on the quintuple nature of the universe. "All things originated from food (annam). We live by food alone, and food is considered as the curing herb. Those who adore Brahman for food receive food. The breath (prana) is all beings ' lives. Those who adorate Brahman as life come to life. Mind (manas) is beyond air, and words can not touch Brahman. Knowledge (vijnana) is beyond mind. As Brahman, all gods adorate Vijnana. Yet Brahman, the root of everything, is beyond Vijnana."

The five layers of personality are described here. The outside layer is the physical body, the second, the electric body (pranamaya kosha) the third layer is the intellectual body (manomaya kosha), the wisdom core, and then the blissful body (anandamaya kosha). the second layer is the electric body. The sage gives us the "calculus of bliss" in order to understand Brahman's bliss: "Let there be a beautiful and well-known youth, who is very strong and very swift, so that the whole universe may become his dominion. This is one unit of joy we must call. The peace of the gandharvas is hundred times the happiness of joy and happiness. The Upanishad continues its hierarchy sequence of ten stages, until he enters the bliss the Indra encounters, then Brhaspati and then Prajapati. The Upanishad continues its Hierarchical sequence of ten stages. Finally, the happiness of Brahman is 1010 times greater than that of the rich, beautiful youth, which has all the wealth of the world. But the joy of a Brahman knower, who is not hit by desire, is the same as that of Brahman."

When we think about ourselves, we tend to think about our own minds or at all. But we should focus on and "eat" another dimension of our personality. We know the wisdom "sheath" or sheet that is very close to the "blissful sheath." The Upanishad therefore teaches that Brahman is not very far away, it is very near.

The Chandogya Upanishad

The name of Upanishad comes from the word chanda, which refers to a poetic meter. The essence of this Upanishad is the importance of language and singing in life, poetically articulated. "Speaking yields milk," she says, as she sets the course of our lives and is the basis of our food. After the "interior singing" in our air system has been pointed out, it underlines that we need to be mindful of it in all our chants and singing. Otherwise it humorously says,' If we do anything' heedlessly,' our head will fall down'.

This is one of the long Upanishads with a variety of tales to describe his lessons. Just as the Mandukya centered on Om, the Upanishad starts as a lute singing with an instruction to meditate on Om. The essence of all beings is earth,' continues,' water is the essence of the world, water is plants ' essence, the plants ' essence is a individual, speech is the meaning of one's being, the Rg Veda is the anthem of speech, the chanting is the essence of the anthem, udgith is the ultimate expression of chant. Om holds talk and breath together.

While the Upanishads teach us that Brahman goes beyond mind and language, they are also trying to tell us that it is similar in every air of our life, closer than nearby in the world around us and. A person's essence is language and how significant that is! What a person thinks, knows, feels in his / her speech is revealed. Breathing is an important factor in chat. The "heart singing" of Om puts speak and air together.

"The light (deva) and the dark (asura) interplay within this body. The gods believed the udgitha was sense of smell, but since we could detect good and evil things, it could not be. Then udgitha, the gods believed, was voice, but since we could say both good and bad words, it can not be. The gods thought udgitha was the sense of vision, but, as we can see good and evil, it couldn't be. Then the gods thought udgitha is sight, but because both good and bad can be heard, it cannot be. Then the gods considered udgitha was mind, but it can't be good or bad as we can imagine. Then udgitha as prana (life) was thought about and the gods realized that prana couldn't be penetrated by the dark.

In this series of verses, we see the student lead to see how everything, good and bad, is filled with duality, and then eventually, the prana is not, and thus we understand a Brahman side like that. Then the gods thought udditha as life (prana) and knew that darkness could not reach prana.

The Upanishad follows other guidelines as to how to meditate on this instruction. "Anyone like udgith should meditate on the sun. The sun knows no darkness just like the udgitha. You can meditate on the breathing like udgitha because it sings Om all the time. The song of the udgitha is like the vina (a stringed instrument). The song is about us too. The track's in the rain. The track is in the rivers. The track is in the seasons. The song is in the birds' and animal's sounds. As the branch holds all the leaves together, so is the whole of Om's speech. It's all Om truly".

The Upanishad's central argument is that "album" is an essential part of life and that the music has to be one. The poetic mood is a way towards a higher consciousness. This perception is knowledge- transcending. "Is one who writes poetry to describe anything in his book" My Reminiscence, "the Bengali poet and Nobel Prize-winner, Rabindranath Tagore? It is a feeling the seeks to find external form in a poem in the brain. There was an error. The only difficulty is that words have meaning. This is why the writers must turn around and change them in meters and in rhymes so that meaning is somewhat tested and can be conveyed.". "The main aim of teaching is not to explain, but to knock at the mental doors. There was a mistake. I can remember a lot of things that I didn't understand but were deeply moving. There was a mistake. Late in the afternoon, I was walking our house's terrace. There has been a mistake. I could see that the night had come through me; I had been washed off by its colors. There has been a mistake. I saw the world in its true nature now that the self was in the past... With Beauty and joy all over."

As the wise man continues, "The heart has five openings. Remembering Prasna Upanishad. The breath is prana, the breath is vyana, the breath is apana, the breath is saman and the breath is udana. You ought to think about it. There was a mistake. Yes, a person is anticipated. It is intended for the purpose."

Here are some excellent examples. A young boy who wanted to know went to a wise person to be taught. The wise man asked him, "What is your dad's name?" The kid answered, "I don't know my dad's name. When my mother served several people, I was born. Then the sage said," Nobody except a brahmin can talk such a damaging truth about oneself. I just know my name is Satyakama and my mother is Jabala. "I will teach you because you did not deviate from reality." An important feature of this time is evident here. The true meaning of Brahmin is a genuine seeker of truth, not a caste difference.

A different way of instructing the sage is now coming. The wise man gives 400 lean cows to Satyakama, to be taken into the forest. Bring them back when they're a thousand. Satyakama then follows orders and one cow talks to him after a few years,' We are a thousand, so bring us back to your teacher. Satyakama was struck and said, "Translate for me, please." The cow replied, "East Brahman, and west Brahman, so I'm telling you about Brahman. Brahman is the north and the south is the same thing. So Satyakama went to the flames, and said," Please teach me, please." Then the Fire said, "Brahman is the world, so is the ocean and the sky. Then Satyakama came and said," Know me! "and the birds said," The sun and moon belong both to Brahman, and also to the lightning. The sun and moon, as it were, are part of the moon. When Satyakama took the cows back to the teacher, the wise man said, "Your face shines as a Brahman-knower. The teacher is Brahman, and so are hearing and sight and mind." Who's been teaching you? The wise man taught him then and nothing was left out. "Beings other than humans, but now I think you can show me.".

Vivekananda writes to us about the voices of cows, fire, birds, etcetera when he describes the significance of this story. "All of the voices inside us are the brilliant concept we see here as a virus. When we better understand these realities, we realize that the voice is in our own heart. There was a mistake. The second idea we have is to obey Brahman's wisdom. The fact was demonstrated by everything the students learned. There was a mistake. The world has been transformed, life has been transformed, the sun, the moon, the stars, the lightning. All those stories are based on the principle that invented symbolism can be good and helpful, but better symbols than anyone we can invent exist. The early thoughtlets spoke to this world. Birds spoke with them; animals were talking to them; the sun and the moon spoke with them and they learned things little by little and became in the center of nature. They did not learn the truth through cogitation, by the power of the reasoning, by selecting other people's brains and creating a great text, as in modern times, not even I did, through taking one of their writings and making a lengthy lecture, but by careful inquiry and exploration. the main method was by practicing and so it has always been. It is to practice first before knowledge.

The next question reminds us of the Mundaka Upanishad's opening question. The student asks, "Master, what does it all mean to learn that?" The sage answered: "This teaching is just as understood through understanding a clod of clay. It would bleed out of this mighty tree, but still live, if anyone struck the root. It would bleed, but still live, if someone were to strike in the middle. Being impregnated with the man it is strong, drinking and cheerful. The student presents it to me, and says, "Sir, it's here." "Break it." "It broke, Sir." "There's a break." "Sir," he says. "What do you see? Sir.' Split one of the grains.'" It's gone, sir." "What you see? What do you see? Sir? "Nothing, sir." "My dear, it great Nyagrodha tree has come forth out of that' nothing.' The atman, from which this entire universe has emerged is intangible, imperceptible."

Then a progressive meditation instruction is given. The sage Narada came to another sage, Sanatkumara, saying: "I studied all the fields of education, literature, science, music, philosophy, and sacred scripture. I've got no peace, however. The revered wise man Sanatkumara responds," What you studied is name only. I have learned from great teachers such as you, that only he who knows himself finds peace. "Think of Brahman's name."

What a great lesson! Note that all that Narada knows does not say is unsuccessful. By asking Brahman to meditate on that, He transforms and defiles it. Narada now asks, "Is anything more than name available?" The wise man responds,' Yeah, there's more talk than name. We know the many branches of learning by voice. Dream about Brahman's voice."

"Is something superior to speech?" This is a question of Narada. "The mind is higher than the words," answers the wise man. Both the word and speak can be held by the mind. "Is anything higher than mind? Meditate on mind, as Brahman." "Narada is asking." It's more will than mind, yes. If you want to, then you think, then you speak, then you utter the word. Thus, as Brahman, meditate on Will." "Is something higher? "Narada's asking." Yes, it's more than will to think. Although you know a lot, but you don't know how to think, you'll say he's nobody, no matter how he knows. Think about Brahman's thinking."

"Has something higher been there, sir?" Narada's concerned. "Indeed, contemplation exceeds thinking. As it were, the earth looks. The sky looks like it is. It looks like the mountains. By contemplation, anyone who has achieved greatness in this world has done so. The contemplation of Brahman requires a separate perception of a series of thoughts.

"Everything higher is there, sir?" Indeed, more knowledge and more understanding. Think about understanding and insight as Brahman. "The patterns arise from detached observations, and that is called the comprehension, that is to say, the perception of a pattern, the" law." "We are more important than knowledge and perspective. Hundred men of understanding will shake a man with both physical and mental energy. The world stands by power, indeed. The mountains stand by power, indeed. The world stands by power, indeed. Meditate on power as Brahman." "Power "here is to be regarded as a lasting effort.

"Nothing better is there, sir?" Food is more powerful than electricity. Neither physical strength or mental strength can be accomplished without nourishment. There is something better, sir? So, meditate on food than Brahman." "Food is greater than nourishment. Food is in Earth, in the soil, in the atmosphere, in the mountains, in the plants and in all life. All these kinds of waters are indeed. "Is there anything higher sir? Then, meditate on food as Brahman." "From food, heat is greater. It won't rain, and there is no water without the convection of heat. Think of Brahman on heat."

"Much higher is there, sir?" There's more room (akasa) than sun. Without room, there can be nothing. Sun, moon and stars lie in space. "That's something higher sir? Meditate on space as Brahman." "There is more space (akasa) than heat. Without space, there can be nothing. The sun, moon and stars lie in space." Is something higher, sir? Think about space as Brahman." "Yeah, more than knowledge, the desire is. Memory will not continue without intention. Memory knows while intoxicated by desire. "Is there anything higher than that, sir? Meditate as Brahman." Indeed, the prana of life is superior to wish. Prana moves breath. Prana moves breath. All this is Prana."

There are some items here that need explanation. We come here to very subtle, interesting thoughts. Through memory, the human memory is not intended, but the universal memory. The hypothesis is that creation takes place through cycles (kalpas) through Indian cosmology. The present universe is destroyed (pralaya), then another universe is formed (or, in reality, a projection). The theory says that the cycle continues cyclically. Where does the new universe live between creation and dissolution? It's in memory. Perhaps like Jung, we will call it the "collective unconscious," but the concept is the same. Where are the archetypes, until we appear in the realms of waking or dreams?

Vivekananda gives some further explanation of these points in his book on cosmology. We are honored. "All motion, all in the world, can be compared to waves that are rising and falling successively. Certain of these philosophers believe that for a time the entire universe settles down. Others argue that this equilibrium is only true for structures ... What becomes of the world when it calms down? It exists in the form of origin, in finer forms only. There was a mistake. There's a lovely passage in the Rg Veda, the oldest human writing ever, and it's most poetical-' If there's neither something, nor nothing, if the darkness rolled over the sky, what lived? What? and it is given the answer,' Then there was a vibration less existence.' Then there was a prana but no motion; anidavatam means existed without vibration.' It'd escaped vibration. When the kalpa stops, the anti-vibrating atom begins vibrating, blowing when prana is given to akasa after blow. The atoms are condensed and various elements are formed as they are condensed. Such things are generally quite strangely interpreted: people don't go to philosophers or writers to explain them and don't have the brains to understand them. A stupid man reads three Sanskrit letters and translates an entire book. If they go to the observers, they will find that it is not air or anything of that sort. They are translated as air, fire, etc. The akasa creates Vayu or Vibrations, works through repeated blows of prana. This Vayu vibrates, and increasing vibrations lead to friction causing hot tejas. Then the fire comes to a halt, apah. This liquid then gets solid. There was a mistake. Everything we know through movement, vibration, or thinking is a prana transition."

Chapter Five

True Experience of The Self Is the Unawareness of Who 'I Really Am'.

When a snake casts out its worn-out skin and then doesn't know it, a person who has discovered it doesn't know his body. If there are no ideas about this universal life of a body-consciousness, suffering and joy, freedom and slavery, etc., disappear and his mind reaches to the fourth stage (Turiya's fourth state). When this state is surpassed by the practitioner, he becomes a Brahman (God) himself and by vague terms, the Upanishads describe the state "Not that." Brahman is not thought.

What is Turiya – The Fourth State of Mind

God is said to be omnipresent. Which means that in every part of your body God lives. There are millions of cells in the body, science claims, each possessing an intellect.

The Four Levels of Consciousness

This implies that God's power resides in each and every cell of the body. But it's resting. In the body lie resting all the gods and goddesses. You're not meditating because of that. Your mind is tight to feed, drink, raise, and tell lies. It has Jag Rita, Swapna and Sushupti. It is tight. You know only about these three consciousness states. You are alive, or you dream, or you sleep.

45

You're not aware of a fourth condition. But in a human being, there is something called Turiya, this is a fourth state, a higher consciousness. The practice of one-pointing of the mind will achieve this higher consciousness. Turiya is the context underlying the three common consciousness states and transcending them. Consciousness is: waking, dreaming and unbelieving sleep.

In verse 7 of the Mandukya Upanishad Turiya is discussed. But in the most ancient Upanishads the term is included. The four states of consciousness are described in Chapters 7.7 through 8.12, for instance, as awake, full of dreams, deep sleep and sleep beyond profound sleep. Brhadaranyaka Upanishad also mentions the state of Turiya in chapter 5.14. Maitri Upanishad talks in sections

6.19 and 7.11 about the fourth state (Turiya).

When during Dhyana one slowly rises above all three states of jagrita, Swapna and Sushupti, and the fresh sky, a fourth state emerges in him. The state in which TURIYA or TURIYA or the fourth condition is that in which the human soul rests in his own Sath Chit Ananda Svarupa.

You should follow these five spiritual practices to reach this fourth state (Turiya).:

Imagine you've got a vision. You bought a plot in that vision and build a house. The house is full and you call the house-warming ceremony your beloved mates. But in the meantime, because of some happening or human you have been awoken from sleep. Though, the dream continues. You send your friends a sumptuous dinner and plan the party together with suitable entertainment facilities like a big host. However, because you're out of your dream, you won't know these occurrences. Now just think of the whole world as a dream for a moment. Now you're awakened for example in the north.

Now you know nothing about what's happening in the world out of your dream. Since no one is seeing the universe now, when you wake up, you don't know or remember what is or was going to happen here. These thoughts offer another kind of mind calm and godly joy.

In the same way, what if we believe that our mind is just like a mirage and the reflector of a pure conscience is in it.? You may know the concept of a mirage in a desert. Mind and ego are not things real; they are superimposed on pure consciousness (like the mirage of the sun's rays). Such reflections are helpful to eradicate our ego.

The practice should always believe that he is about 10-20 feet away from his body. He needs only to believe he's a body witness. The practitioner has no experience of physical suffering, enjoyment, honor or dishonor. In this state. In times of even the biggest and most extreme miseries and misfortunes His mind remains cool and happy. He is truly peaceful.

Only imagine if you stand before an anthill. The ants run with great enthusiasm here and there are maize spikes in their mouths. You meet each other at any moment, yet you can not cross any small stream of water.

Anthill

Some hobbies you may think are stupid because you aren't an ant. Seek to be a superman in the same way to look at the world. Then you will know that all glory, abundance of money, cities, and so on are infantile like the ants. That's why your mind is a spiritual mind now. You will always feel Spiritual Joy through practicing of this spiritual practice. your appetite for worldly pleasures and hobbies will diminish.

Think highly of the god Almighty leading and guiding all acts in this world. There is nothing if he and his symbols are not noticed. You will consider your life and acts to be controlled by it as you are a minute part of the universe. Your lives are formed by His will. Trust is central in this reasoning. This is not fatalism but a fact. You will believe that lifting your hands is His will and not yours. At an advanced stage of this spiritual practice, the meaning of the self is totally annihilated and the practitioner is persuaded that his will governs the acts of this world and his body. You can begin to think you're a marionette ruled by Almighty god. Your life is bound to become godly, healthy and glorious under his leadership. Such spiritual rituals should not be conducted like other meditations in a sitting position and at a fixed time.

Dreaming is not only Dreaming; it's true, it's important. For explanations, you can't dream. There's a causality even of a dream. It's significant, it tells you something. Instead, it tells more about you and reveals more when you're big, because if you're waking you and others can deceive yourself and others, but you can't disappoint your dreams. Dreams are harder because we have not yet found a system for dreaming and dreaming with masks. The dreams are still naked, genuine; they show more truly the real face when you are awake than anyone you use.

And, this paradoxical thing that can happen: a dream becomes true, because you don't handle it, you don't– you're hilflose. You're true. A vision occurs; there is nothing you can do. You're not the doer, you can only be the watchman. You are completely helpless in a subtle manner. Due to this impotence, your dream gets real, genuine and reveals much about your mind. Vision is valuable to know and to ask. The UPANISHAD then asks, "What is this awake mind state? What is it that dreams? What's sleep that doesn't dream? And TURIYA is what it is?"

This term "turiya" only means "the fourth," and what is the fourth thing to be able to overcome all these three – alive, dreaming, deeply asleep? The fourth wasn't named; only the fourth, the turiya, was recognized because that is simply not a state of the mind, but of one's own existence.

During the whole day, you will revolve the above thoughts. Finally, you can believe that this world view is just an Almighty sport. He won't take any misfortune, deceit, embarrassment, etc. he could be subjected to seriously. Spiritual practice number five is supreme among all of the above five spiritual practices and produces fast results to the fourth (Turiya) state.

Chapter Six

Meditation

One is analyzing an item, dividing it into its pieces, but not all pieces. They are the whole item,

but they don't suit the whole thing. Without the parts, the whole can't be formed. But the whole thing is more, more than all the elements combined. The mystery is something more.

Science is divided and the effects of the information are analyzed. The opposite aspect is faith. Religion believes in integration, not separation. Religion continues to add, to sum up. And when all is done– nothing is out, all is included, and this whole is seen, taken as a whole– the divine appears. And science can never claim there's a deity– it's unlikely. No one can expect science to say there's a god any day, because the very method of analysis can't lead to the whole. The cycle itself leads to the smallest part– never the whole– because it relies on division.

Research can never come into the world, into being, to any divinity, because divinity is something that comes from the whole. It's not math; it's organic. It's not electric, it's real. Then put them back, but I won't be found there. They can break me into parts. But I am not a mechanical device, I am not just parts stowed up and organized. You put everything in its place again. More than all pieces, something is there– something is missing.

Life by analysis can never be understood. Only the material, never the spiritual can know analyzes. These are the two intelligence dimensions. If anyone assumes, though, that there is nothing but matter, it just means he's used the empirical approach– nothing else. When somebody says nothing, but only knowledge, this only means that he used the process of synthesis– not analysis. Freud used analysis as a methodology; he could not understand then that in man there was any spirit, any spiritual dimension. But a second psychologist, Assagioli, uses synthesis now as his method.: It's not a body, just the mind, just consciousness. Whenever someone affirms matter or understanding, it indicates that a certain search process has been used. Analysis is logic– Passion is synthesis.

This is why religion was always illogical, and science always charming. The creation of the ego is to be associated as something you are not. The ego means the something you are not marked as. Either way, no tag is needed. You don't have to be associated: you are. So, every time there is a tag, it means that you're not with something else. The body and the mind can be marked. Nevertheless, as soon as you are associated, you are lost. That's the essence of the ego. This is the creation and crystallization of Ego. When you say "I," something is in description– with name, shape, body, history, mind, thought, memory. I'm a supporter. It's a profound appreciation, you can only say I. If you don't know anything else and will live with yourself, you won't say I; I just drops down. You can't say I. "I" is description meaning.

Identity is the cornerstone of all slavery: be acquainted and you are in jail. The prison is going to be the very identity. Don't be marked, stay completely yourself, otherwise independence remains. This is slavery, therefore: Ego is tyranny, so ego is liberty. And this ego is nothing but something you are not acquainted with. All are marked with their names, for example; and all born with no names. The name then becomes so critical that one can die for the sake of his name.

What is a name? What is a name? But it becomes very important as soon as you are remembered. And without a name– nameless, everybody is born. Or, you take shape; everyone has his own shape marked. You stand in front of your mirror every day. What do you see? What do you see? – You yourself? – Yourself? No, not that. No mirror may represent YOU, just the shape with which you are marked. But this is the foolishness of the human mind, that the shape is constantly changing every day and never is you disappointed. What was your shape when you were a child?? How was your form when you were in the womb of your mother? What was your shape when you were planted by your parents? Would you remember the egg in the womb of your mother if an image is made for you? Would you understand and say, "I'm that?" No, but with this egg somewhere back, you must have been marked... You were born– and if you can recreate the first scream for yourself, will you remember so say,' This is MY scream?' Indeed, but it was yours, and you must be honored.

If a dying man can create an album.... The type is constantly changing– consistency remains, but always a transition.... Every seven years the body completely, completely changes; nothing, not a single cell, remains the same. We think now, "this is my shape, this is me," but perception is unformed. The form is something else that changes, changes and changes– just like clothing.

It is an ego that decides this. If you don't know anything– names, or forms, or anything– what's the ego? You're suddenly, and yet you aren't. Then you are completely pure, but you have no ego. This's why Buddha called the self, no-self; he said, "There's no ego, you can't call yourself ATMA, just ANATTA." That's why he called the self. The pure life is independence. You should call yourself' I;' there's no' I.' It can't really be translated this word AVIDYA. Not ignorance; it's not stupidity... It's not ignorance... Since indifference is only negative. You don't know, you're stupid.

But it's not a negative thing, it's very hopeful. You don't know anything, but you know something that isn't. You say something that isn't. Rather, this avidya is a positive picture of something that is not. The "I" is not– the ego is the world's most non-existent.

It looks really important and is entirely empty. Avidya means this ego, this image of yourself, as the projective source inside you. Avidya is in you a projective power. It's not ignorance only; it's not something that you don't know; you can construct something that isn't. You can dream something you can't, imagine something you can't. If the mind constructs something that's not, it's avidya. This way of removing all projections and all identifying things is called vidya when this mind removes all projections, and all that is not, it seems to be, remains without any projective operation. Vidya is not intellect. Again, vidya is a good force for destruction of everything that creates avidya. Vidya can't be traduced. Vidya is a positive force in you that can destroy the development of ego. They're both positive: avidya creates what isn't and vidya kills what isn't. So vidya is yoga, vidya is religious science.

And what does it actually mean to us as Yoga, Ayurveda, or meditation?

The first thing to understand is that our Yoga sadhanas or spiritual path is not literally a waking self. It is part of our inner self which existed before this corps was born and continues past its end.

This interpretation of the four states and the self-witness behind them demonstrates that our waking life is a dream, too. We've got two dream states, so to speak. The first is a dream state, that is our own individual minds ' personal and subjective vision. The second, the waking status that we share with many other individuals, is a mutual and rational vision.

And our entire lives are more than just a night. There's a lot we don't know, though we know other things in life. Especially the essence of our very being, or the actual meaning of the existence, we do not know. Our minds and senses only provide us with a superficial and limited awareness of duality, mistake and ignorance. The darkness, ignorance and lack of knowledge of deep sleep often affect the waking and the dream state. Our waking mind is wrapped in darkness, unaware who we are, why we were born, when our consciousness emerged and what will happen to us after our death.

We are usually concerned with and never look behind the physical body, awakening, waking ego. Obviously, this waking state concentrates in a powerful way on biological, psychological and social needs. It is mainly in terms of the impulses of the wakeful state even when we become more conscious. We forget that behind and beyond waking, dreaming and deep sleep is the eternal Dreamer of our true Soul.

For meditators, the most important consideration of understanding the four consciousness states is that this is not only through the waking, but also via the dream and deep sleep that we should establish our meditation. We not only should seek to promote the interests of the self of the ego, but also of the Self of the four nations. Above all, we should address the concerns of our immortal soul, that takes birth in many bodies and worlds.

Meditation will awaken the true reality and perpetual state of the Divine Awakening, the everlasting day of clear light of consciousness, from the universal dream. Meditation should be an inquiry into the wake, dream, deep sleep and beyond, and it should continue every second, 24 hours a day.

To do our meditation is an important means to turn dream and sleep into meditation. It is the latest procedure before night. Those who night in meditation are what was called yoga nidra or yogic sleep in which we are consciously sleepy as a way to absolute transcendence. Deep meditation is, indeed, much like entering a deep sleep during the waking state, removing the consciousness from the mind and body. We should see that sleeping at night is the chance for deep meditation over and above all world illusions.

In short, note that your everyday step from waking to deep sleep to dreaming is a Spiritual journey into consciousness, an awareness that you can unlock the mysteries of cosmic consciousness within yourself. Every day is a beautiful chance to learn yourself. You only live at a time of one day. But everyday is paradise when you do so, every day is love, every day is full of happiness.

How to encourage people during meditation. The best way The first thing: You must make it clear that the patient is sick to go to the hospital, otherwise the hospital will not have to go. The people that you wish to encourage in meditation must first tell them they are disappointed, maybe for too long, that they are sad. If you laughed from your very heart, you can not remember. They've become robots –so they have to be done, but they have no pleasure. They live a life of tragedy. Your birth is accidental, your marriage is by accident, your children are by accident, your work is by accident. There is no sense of growth and orientation in their lives. That's why they can't be happy.

So, you must first make them aware of their circumstance- and almost everyone is in the same place. Death is drawing near- you can't trust yourself to be here tomorrow. And your life is a complete desert- no oasis has been found, no purpose, no importance has been felt- and death will ruin all future possibilities. So, you must first let them know their pointless, unintended, irritated lives. We know it, but we try to suppress their knowledge in many ways, because to know it constantly is torture. So, they go to the movies to forget it. They go to festivals, they go to picnics, they drink alcoholic beverages; they do everything- just to somehow not realize the truth of their lives, their hollowness, their futility.

This is the main part- to remind you. And once a person remembers all that, it's very easy to lead them into meditation, since meditation is the only answer to all man's questions. It can be anger, disappointment, sorrow, meaninglessness, anguish: there may be a lot of problems, but the solution is one thing.

Meditation is the answer.

And the simplest meditation form is only a way to bear witness. There are a Hundred and Twelve meditation techniques, but experiencing is an important part of a Hundred and Twelve methods. Experiencing is the only way, as far as I am concerned. Those a Hundred and Twelve are different witnesses ' applications. The secret, the meditative spirit, is to know how to witness.

You see a tree: you've come, it's the tree, but you can't find one more thing? - you see the tree, there's a proof inside you that you see the tree. The universe is not divided into the object and the subject alone. There is something beyond both, and beyond that there is meditation. So, in all the acts... And for an hour or half an hour in either the morning or the evening, I don't want people to sit. This kind of meditation will not improve because if you meditate for an hour, you do the reverse for 23 hours.

Meditation can be victorious: it can spread across 24 hours a day by observing.

Do not eat with the server, mark yourself. There's the fridge, the fridge is there, and you sit here. Only walk, let your body go, only look. The knack is coming, slowly. It's a blowjob and you can once see little things....

Crowing this crow... You're listening. You're listening. Those two are object and subject. However, you can't see a witness who sees both of you? –The crow, the listener, and there's always someone who looks at the two. The phenomenon is so plain. You can then move deeper: you can look at your thoughts and your emotions, your moods. You can see your feelings. No need to say,' I'm sad.' Indeed, you are a witness of the passage of a cloud of sadness. You can just be a witness, There's wrath. You never get upset– you don't have a way to get angry– you always are a witness. You're not always angry. You're just a mirror; the rage comes and goes. Things occur, reflect, shift– and the reflections hold the mirror empty and clean, scratch less.

Finding your inside mirror is witnessing.

And once you've found it, wonders begin to take place. Thoughts disappear as you actually observe the thoughts. Then unexpectedly you never knew a profound silence. When you watch people's moods, rage, sorrow, happiness, suddenly they vanish and there is even more silence. And then the revolt when there's nothing to watch. Then the attention of the witness turns to himself, because it can not be stopped, no object is left. It's a beautiful word ' do.' It just means that you do not, you object. If your witness is not object, he simply returns to himself– to the source. And it is at this point that one becomes very enlightened.

Meditation is just a journey: the result is ever a Buddhahood. And learning this time is knowing everything. There's then no pain, no disappointment, no lack of meaning; life's not an accident, though. It's an essential part of this cosmic whole. And a great joy emerges from the need of you for this whole life. The need for man is greatest. You feel gratified if someone needs you. But if you need all of your life, your happiness will not be constrained. And even a little grass blade is needed for this life like the biggest star. Inequality is not at issue. No one can replace you. Unless you are there, life will always be something less and something less– it never will be complete. The feeling— that all of this incredible life needs you — removes from you all miseries. You came home for the first time.

The Night Meditation

This evening meditation, without opening my eyes, will be a continuous star at me for thirty minutes. Just take thirty minutes to look at me. See your eyes like bars, and your consciousness comes to me from those bars. Go forward with the impression that your mind is reaching me, and do not open your eyes. This continuous gazing produces a very profound mutation in the bio energy, the kundalini, the spinal energy, the strength of the serpent. Go on jumping for 30 minutes. Your hands shall be lifted up in heaven as though you were rising to Heaven. When your hands are lifted, you're going to have to look at me and you're going to have to run and start using the chant, the chant of "hoo." –It's an unimportant tone. This "hoo" is just like a hammering inside the spinning air, so that the snake starts to move upwards. You are beginning to feel a subtle air stream in your spine; energy is rising and rising. You are going to be weightless.

"Always use the mantra for 30 minutes!" Woo! Woo! Hoo! Huh! Huh! "Jumping, looking at me with intensity.... Then I'll tell you to stop thirty minutes, and lie down, dead, ten minutes. It's the experiment at night. We're going to do a new meditation tomorrow morning. Everything we have done this morning, today, will be done in the evening. Instead of a silent meditation, kirtan meditation is done in the afternoon. And we'll do a four-step meditation in the morning. The first phase, a short breath of 10 minutes– so quickly that your body is oxidized energy. Then a catharsis for 10 minutes. Just throw it out, whatever happens inside you. Go and dance, weep, make noise, laugh, weep– be free to express it, whatever you feel. Then the "hoo" mantra will be used for 10 minutes in the third step. And then in the fourth step, absolutely rest for thirty minutes, as though you died.

That's going to be tomorrow's morning meditation. And the afternoon meditation of today's morning will be used from 4 to 5. And this exercise, which we will do now, will be continued throughout the camp throughout the night. So now we continue the exercise at night.

Chapter Seven

Yoga, Meditation on Om, Tapas, And Turiya In the Principal Upanisads.

In his Meditation, Yoga, and Freeth treatise, Mircea Eliade starts by saying that the center of Indian spirituality is directly linked through four basic and interdependent principles, four film concepts. It's karma, Maya, meditation, nirvana. The other three would obviously have to be discussed A coherent history of Indian philosophy could be written from any one of these basic concepts. With respect to the creation of yoga during the Principal Upanisads time, I propose that Yoga, Om syllable meditation, Om tapas and Turiya are equally interdependent, and that analyzes of one of them directly lead to analysis of the other three. The Maitri Upanisads sum up these ideas, but they are also discussed in previous Upanisads. In the Matri Upanisad, we find the statement that the meditation on the syllable Om is the way to make the practitioner aware of samadhi. This book briefly explores the development of yogic practices from Vedic sacrifices to their current manifestation in Western hatha yoga and analyzes the principal Upanisads in order to investigate the internalization of ancient external communal sacrifice fire rituals. Tapas, which culminate in the fourth state of consciousness, turiya, and one of the main forms of Yoga and

Tapas, becomes the common thread that winded through the tradition of yogic activities, meditation on the syllable Om.

The name yoga is derived from the root yuj and is used to bind, hold or yoke together. It means that the body, mind, spirit and spiritual must be unified or united; it may be interpreted as the atman and brahman's unity in terms of Vedanta. The oldest known shape is the controlled or meditative approach of Yoga in combination with sacrificial rituals.1 However the traditions of ancient rsis are better known to us as the tapás. Yoga seems to date to the Vedas. Yoga seems to have been in its oldest known shape. The earliest name for yoga-like traditions in India is tapas Feuerstein. This old Sanskrit word simply means fire.... In the Rig-Veda the word is sometimes used to describe the qualities and function of the solar orb (God Surya) or the fire of the sacrifice (or God Agni), as its own deity. In such situations, the heat of the sun and fire is often expressed in its burning intensity. It is awkward and distressing. In this we can see the source of the subsequent metaphor of the tapas in form of anger and aggression as mental heat but also as fervor, zeal or painting.

Thus, the term tapas have been extended by austerity to the religious or spiritual challenge of voluntary self-discipline.

Feuerstein goes on to suggest that austerity and asceticism are also extremely metaphysical. B. K.

S. Iyengar adds to this tapas concept by saying that tapas are derived to flame, smoking, sparkling, painful or heat-consuming from the root tap sense. It therefore means a smoking effort to achieve a definite purpose in life under all circumstances. It requires bathing, control and discipline... Tapas is the aware effort to attain absolute union with the Divine and to branch out all passions that impede this purpose.

Kaelber's examine the transition of tapas from the Vedic to the Upani-sads, in contrast to the tapas of meditation which seek to realize the Brahman, proposes a distinction between 2 types of tapeas, namely tapas of outer rituals of sacrifice and duties such as almsgiving. Kaelber notes that this distinction has been established in reincarnation Upanisads. This means that sacrificial tapas (which he calls low tapas) are devalued and human transcendental tapas (that he calls high tapas) are more emphasized in Upanisads. The tapas revered in the principal Upanisads are different forms between tapas, identified with a clear knowledge between truth itself, not with traditional sacrifices, but rather with meditation. Also, Kaelber notes that tapas (is) are increasingly related to inaction less meditation and mental focus. î6 Further, Kaelber stresses that tapas are the means and end because Brahman's understanding or knowledge removes any distinction of subject and object.: By way of Tapas and knowledge one knows the tapas and knowledge of Atman / Brahman itself. The sources of knowledge are one with the known entity. The meditative tapas of the ascetic are not merely a way of understanding the ultimate reality; they are the ultimate reality itself.

Deussen claims that all that is good is dependent on tapas in the world... The emperor protects his kingdom through tapas, the gods are fleeing death. One way of doing tapas is meditation on Om's syllable, as we will see in our analysis of the Upanisads. Similar to Kaelber's above equation of tapas and last-reality, Brahman, we will see how the primordial sound Om and yoga and meditation-related breathing are linked with final reality. In the time of the Upanisads, we shall focus on internalizing the yogic practices. The Upanishadic wise men overwhelmingly turned to meditative practice, or internal worship (Upasana), the main way to receive transcendental wisdom, as Feuerstein says. Conversely, orthodox brahmins continued to practice meditation intimately connected to sacrificial rituals. Although the goal-to transcend ordinary consciousness

and profound truth, Maya-remained the same, the means and emphasis during the Upanisads changed dramatically. Specifically, yoga can be seen as internalized asceticism in a certain way. Where the former ascetic still stands under the burning sun to win deity's favor, yogin or yogini's work takes place mainly in his or her own consciousness ' laboratory. Hume echoes this when he says that the last solution to the practical problem offered by the Upanishads, that is to say the Yoga, is the product of the idea of strict unity that started the Upanishad hypothesis that urged them from cosmology to intellectual monism and from external to inner unity.

The relationship between tapas and the realization of unity developed during the Upanisads is turiya. As we see from both the Upanisads, Mandukya and Maitri, the fourth (that) is unfathomable, without a distinctive marc, unimaginable and unknown to be name is four stages of consciousness: awake, sleeping, dreaming and the fourth. Drive. Mand. Mand. Deussen states that the disappearance of the consciousness of objects and union with the everlasting intellectual subject created by yoga is the 4th state of man on the wake-up dream and deep sleep of the world. It is exemplified by the Aumkara, its A-U-M parts, the waking, the dreaming, and the sleeping phases, Radhakrishnan said. It is not an exclusive self, but the core of everyone, their personality. Therefore, yoga as philosophical system grows in Upanisads via tapas that evolve to internalize and focuses on meditation on the sacred sound of Om; in effect, the sacred sound Om leads us to a highest level of consciousness, turiya.

The officialization of yoga as a darsana or viewpoint by Patanjali preceded the core Upanisads. Nevertheless, the Yoga Upanisads are distinct from the Yoga sutras of Patanjali. The union-metaphor, as conceived by Patanjali in the second century C.E., does not in any way fit with the classical yoga method. There is no mention of a union with the transcendental truth as the ultimate target of the yogic effort in Patanjali Yoga Sutras (the fundamental scripture of classical yoga). The primary objective in yoga is for Patanjali, as Patanjali says at the beginning of the Yoga Sutras, to avoid the variations of ordinary states. Writes Eliade: The goal of Patanjali Yoga, therefore, is to eliminate two essentially logically and metaphysically mistaken types of perceptions, and to replace them with a sublime, supra-sensory and alien experience. Via samadhi, the yogin finally passes forever over the human condition-dramatic, suffering and painful-and finally enjoys the total freedom the Indian soul longs so ardently for.

The Samkhya is distinct from Yoga: first of all, Patanjali's yoga is theistic, revering a supreme Lord. Additionally, though the only path to salvation according to Samkhya is spiritual knowledge, yoga has put significant emphasis on meditation techniques. Eliade makes a stronger distinction by suggesting that Yoga, like Samkhya's, is intended to abolish a normal consciousness in favor of the nature of a particular consciousness which can fully understand the metaphysical reality. Even, with yoga, it is not so easy to remove natural consciousness. In addition to the theory, Darsana, it also requires a process (abhyasa), an asceticism (tapas).

The Bhagavad Gita, who Feuerstein certainly finds to be the most popular yoga player came after Patanjali and the Yoga Upanisads. Then in the fifteenth century, inspired by the Tantra and Buddhism, the hatha yoga tradition started. But the intention remains similar to the tapas of the Vedic sacrifices: the experience of ecstatic union takes place in the incarnated State as observed by Feuerstein. Therefore, the hatha yogin seeks to strengthen the body -to bake it.

Before I go into a study of the Principal Upanisads, I will conclude by noting that the focus in hatha yoga practice today continues in the West on tapas or heat generation in the body. Even though the religious or spiritual aspects are rarely mentioned, hatha yoga now generally warms the spine by welcoming the light, producing heat by motion and manipulating opposites. This will be further discussed in our study of the Maitri Upanisads.

While the Katha Upanisad is often considered to be the old Upanishad, who deals with yoga directly. Firstly, before focusing on the Katha, Svetasvatar, Mundaka, Mandukya, and Maitry Upanisad, we'll look at Brhadaranyaka, Chandogya, Taittiriya, Aitareya, Kausitaki, and Kena Upanisads briefly.

Brhadaranyaka Upanisad

It is deemed to be the earliest Upanisad in Brhadaranyaka. The cosmological elements of the sacrificial horse ritual are primarily involved. The horse sacrifice was a significant ritual in honor of a powerful king to ensure that his rule continued success. The sacrifices mentioned in the Brhadaranyaka Upanisads are reminders of the history and evolution of yoga, but more importantly, the supremacy of breath is emphasized in the physical functions of Kaelber. The Brhadaranyaka Upanisad, the breath of the many gods is deified: Yajnavalkya reduces all 3306 gods to one god following discussion:

Who is the one god?

He told Air. Brahma, the Yon (tya) they call it.

Later, after a debate on Atman, BU 6.1.7 breath proves very powerful over all other components and functions of the body. For without voice, eyes, ears, mind or semen the body will live, but without breath.

Chandogya Upanisad

The Chandogya Upanisad stresses also the importance of air, like the Brhadaranyaka Upanisad. The Fifth Prapathaka again shows that a breath is indeed the leading and the strongest of all vital breaths, because it is impossible to avoid it that the other vital breaths are obliged to know that the breath is superior. The emphasis in the Chandogya Upanisad on Om is however more important to the development of yoga. The Chandogya Upanisad begins with a chant discussion and forms the connection between speech and respiration which is more evident in the Om syllable. The explanation for this is because Brahman is both Om and Air. The primordial sound here is related to that essential feature of man, air.

Om is also considered by Prajapati as the whole universe: Prajapati has incubated the cosmos and the triple Veda has arisen from these. He incubated the triple Veda, and the syllables of bhur, bhuvar and svar were incubated. Those syllables he incubated, and the syllable Om came forth from them when they had been incubated. Since all the leaves have a pine bored, Om bore all of the words. All this world is only Om.

With regard to what later in Maitri Upanisads as Yoga will synthesize, Chandogya Upanisad is essential given the weight imposed on the sacred syllable Om.

The Khuas, atman and Brahman are later on equal in the Treceeth and Fourteenth centuries, and this time by light: here in the distance above, there is the light shinning from Heaven on the back of everything, at the back of all things, in the highest of the highest worlds. Here we realize that the last one resides within one another and the last one is the entire world; thus, there is harmony between the entire world and one another. But the topic of light inside is even more important for our study of the nature of Yoga: it is visualized– if you feel the heat here in the body through touch.

It is heard when you close your ears and hear a sound, as if that were a flame, as though it were a burning fire. You must value the light as something seen and heard.

Here we see the internalization of the flames of the Vedic Rites of the Sacrifice as this omnipresent light warms the body. While Yoga is not mentioned here, the theory on which Yoga is based is obviously a precedent.

Taittiriya Upanisad

There is a lot of discussion in the Taittiriya Upanisad that solves food; everything seems to be regarded as food (anna). However, Feuerstein says that the very first unequivocal instance of the word yoga seems to be the stimulation of the sage's fickle senses in the scientific sense as in this scripture (2.4.1, p. 2). In 2.4.1, the right side is to be the faith (sraddha): the right side is to be the head; the correct side is the left side; meditation (yoga), body is to take hold; the strength (mahas); the lower part is to be the base. This is to be seen in 2.4. 1..

Aitareya Upanisad

The Aitareya Upanisad is a short journey, mainly concerned with the creation of the worlds from oneself. There are no specific references with regard to yoga and tapas. However, Radhakrishnan says of the Aitareya Upanisad that it is the purpose of the Upanisad to lead the victim's mind to its inner meaning from the external ceremonial. Any real sacrifice is internal.

Kausitaki Upanisad

Ironically, Kausitaki Upanisad compares Breath (prana) with Brahma in 2.1. Upanisad says, "Honestly, honestly, truly, the mind(mana) is the messenger, the eye, the watcher; the voice, the preacher; the speech, the slave." Then in 3.2 the Upanisad explains life and breath: life is the spirit to breathe. The respiratory spirit is truly life, and then it states that one receives immortality with prana which is a logical conclusion that Brahman is eternal.

Kena Upanisad

The Kena Upanisad is a very short, interesting Upanisad because it emphasizes Brahman's basic unknowability, as well as tapas. As far as Brahman is concerned, it says, "There's no eye; there's no voice or mind." We don't know, we don't understand how to tell it. It is other than that which is known, and above that which is unknown.

The Upanisad ends with certain concrete directions after the discussion of Brahman: discipline (tapas), constraint (Dama) and work (Carman) is the cornerstone of this (i.e. the spiritual doctrine). All its founders are the Vedas. His dwelling place is truth. He who knows it (that is, the sacred doctrine) is thus created, striking away evil (papman), in the most wonderful, inexhaustible universe, in the celestial realm.

Katha Upanisad

The Katha Upanisad is the first Upanisad to talk about Yoga in particular. The Katha Upanisad marks the transition from post-Vedic esotericism of the oldest Upanishadstopre-Classically

Yoga of the epic period, according to Feuerstein. Yoga became an authentic tradition with this work. Death says, through the Yoga analysis of what concerns themselves, the sage lets joy and sorrow behind KA U 2.12 The Upanisad then talks about Om as a resource for Brahman because in reality it is Brahman; The Death speaks to Naciketas.

This word is rehearsed by all Vedas and declared by austerities. I would like to describe the word briefly to you, which people live the life of religious studies. It's Om! Om. In truth, Brahma, is that syllable! In addition, this syllable is the highest! To know that syllable, in fact, whatever one wants is his! KA U 2.16-17.

After considering atman and the Naciketa sacrificial fire as an aid, the Upanisad defines the flexibility of the senses, which it renders similar to wild or vicious animals. He, however, who has understanding, whose mind is always held firm, His senses are under control, Like the strong horses of a chariot-driver.

Those who can not control the senses are doomed to reincarnation, samsara. Here the synthesis of the previous Upanisads starts: the Katha Upanisad defines our ontological level and provides us with a way to overcome the state. It also encourages us to take on such a quest, i.e. not to be reborn. Ultimately, when five thoughts are quiet with the mind, reason is not even at work; it is called the highest level, Yoga is summed up as follows.

The Yoga is the way people think when the senses are fully incorporated into it. A man is then free of distractions, as Yoga is the coming and the ceasing being. KA U 6.10 Eliade notes that the Katha is especially important because it emphasizes immortality, freedom from the death, and this is possible only for a person who can control his senses.

Mundaka Upanisad

The Upanisad Mundaka is fascinating because both tapas and Om are being debated. The important value of tapas is founded by Mundaka 1.8: Brahma is built up by austerity. From that food, life- breading, mind, reality, worlds and immortality, also in plays, is created. EOLBREAK Hume translates tapas into austerity, in this passage and Olivelle translates them into fire. In relation to the evolution of yogic practice, both interpretations are viable. Nevertheless, the tapas here render Brahman; Brahman is born of tapas. It is interesting to note. So, for the yoga practitioner, we understand the importance of tapas-or heat production-.

Besides Mundaka Upanisad, which deals with two birds, Om is the second most frequently quoted line. The sacred Om is the bridge. The soul's spear. The symbol of the untraveled man is said to be Brahma, that he must penetrate. It should be like the spear (in the symbol). Mind U 2.2.4.

Mandukya Upanisad

The Mandukya Upanisad is important because it clearly develops the concept of turiya and the relation between the four states of consciousness and Om. Eliade states that the Mandukya marks the triumph of a long labor of synthesis - that is, the integration of several levels of reference: Upanisadic, yogic, mystical cosmological. The Upanisad begins with the mystical word Om being identified with time-Brahman: Om! - This syllable is the whole world... Om, all is the term past, the present and the future. Mand 1 Om, which represents its three components A, U, M and a fourth that exceeds the sum of the pieces, is essential to Upanisadic thinking. Iyengar addresses the implications of the Om syllable,

The letters A, U, and M symbolize the spoken word, the mind and the breath of life (prana) respectively, while the full symbol stands for the living spirit, which is only part of the light of God... Such symbols systematically represent a gunatite that is above and beyond the gunas, and they represent the three gunas or attributes of satva, rajas and tamas. The letters are the 3 time periods– past, current and future– while the whole symbol is the Creator, who transcends the time limits... The A, U and M show the three phases, Asana, pranayama, and prayahara, of yogic discipline. The whole symbol is samadhi, which is the purpose of the three stages.

The fourth symbolism in the atman-brahman, the four-fold division, opens up the way for a daring homology; the four-state consciousness are associated with the four-quarter of the atmen-brahman,

the four elements of om, and when the remarks of Sankara are included, the four yugas. The Mandukya then outlines four consciousness stages, namely, wake, dream, sleep and the fourth. The next line, therefore Om is the Self (Atman), even though Eliad believes that the connection between turiya, the fourth state of consciousness, and Om is, as inferred by Mandukya 12, the connection between us humans as well as our understanding of brahman, as the following is defined without the aspect with which there can not be any dealing, the creation cessation, benign, without a second mand U 12. For Indians, the ultimate goal of all responsible lives is, he writes, total reintegration– that is, a return to unity. This is expressed in Feuerstein's debate on the Mandukya when he says what this Yoga means is the progressive and not dualist practice of the Self, without the so-called objective world touch or interference. He continues to say that Turiya can always be done that the mind has to give up the illusion of a multiplicity of the universe beyond itself, instead of rest in Selfhood.

Svetasvatara Upanisad

The Upanisad of Svetasvatara addresses samsara release through yoga, meditation and tapas. Eliade believes that no other trait is more widely communicated between divine knowledge and immortality. Svetasvatara is the all-pervading Atman, if we look after him with true austerity (tapas). In Svetasvatara. Before the rules and results of yoga were explicitly defined for the first time, the importance of calming the mind and quieting the vital forces are stated.:

8.By holding his body secure, with the three (upper parts) erected and the senses reach the heart with the mind, a wise man should go over with the Brahma-boat all the streams of fear.

9.When you have repressed your respirations in your body and tested your movements, you can breathe in your nose, like a cart of fearsome horses, and keep your wisdom undistracted.

10.In a clear spot without shaking, heat, and gravel in the sound of water and other propensities Fun for meditation, not offensive to the eye, one should practice Yoga in a hidden retreat sheltered from the wind.

11.The preliminary manifestations of the Brahma in Yoga are rain, rain, smoke, sun, wind, fire flies, lightning, crystal and a moon.

12.   If the fifth quality of yoga is made, it comes from earth, water, fire, air and space, no illness, no aging, no death, he Who has gotten a body from the fire of yoga.

13.　　Lightness, fitness, happiness, facial clearness and enjoyment of voice, odour sweetness and scanty excretions are the first step in the development of Yoga, they say.

14.　　Even as a light tainted by dust shines brightly when cleansed, so when he sees the soul essence (Atman), he is unified, his end is reached and he is released from sorrow.

15.　　When a yoga practicer looks at the essence of the human like a sun, Brahma, Unborn, unborn, unbound, free from all things, by knowing God (Deva).! S U 2. 8-15

For our purposes, the lines of this first important step are like a chariot with vicious horses and body made of the fire of Yoga, and one should breathe through one's noses with reduced breath. Here you can see the role of tapas and the location of tapas. Feuerstein notes that Upanisad Shvetashvatara advises meditation through the offering of the holy syllable om called pranava. The cycle of meditation is described as some sort of churning through which the inner fire is kindled that leads to a manifestation of the glory of the Self. In this context, we must also note the focus on the correct posture, which in the Maitri and later discussions of hatha Yoga evolution will become even more important in relation to asanas. In the end, the effects of yoga are also particularly remarkable when you still engage in samsara cycles, namely, smoothness, fitness, relaxation, clearness of face, good odor and voice and small excretions.

Maitri Upanisad

The Maitri Upanisad summarizes all earlier Upanisadic Yoga, Tapas, Om and Turiya meditation. It starts with a talk of the Vedic fires: what was (only) the formation of (sacrificial fires) for the ancients was truthfully a sacrificial sacrifice to Brahma. Therefore, the sacrifice will meditate on the Soul (Atman) with the formation of those sacrificial flames. MA U 1.1 We see in this sense the internalization of external tapas, the sacrificial fire is transformed into the fire of yoga, and we then see the importance of tapas and meditation. It's Brahma's room! He says who is constantly meditating, completely consumed. While Brahma is apprehended by wisdom (vidya), abstinence (tapas) and meditation (cinta). MA U 4.4.

In the beginning, awareness (vidya) was emphasized more than tapas or meditation but the values of the tapas and of Meditation increased to match those of vidya during the time of the Maitri Upanisads. Tapas and meditation are just as important for Brahma's realization.

Then is echoed the essence of the holy syllable Om: two kinds of brahma are surely: the formed and the formless. Now the formed is unreal; the unformed is reality, the brahma is brightness. It is the formed. This is the same brightness as the light. Truly, Om as their soul (atman) came into being. He split himself three times (atmanam). Om consists of three units of prose (a+u+m). Via them, the entire world is woven, twisted and woven. For so it was said: You can take in yourself and meditate on Om as the light. MA U 6.3

This section is very fascinating as the sun, which also produces heat and could be regarded as the primordial source or the root of tapas, is equal to light-similar to the light described in the Chandogya Upanisads. Brahman is the sun that is the light, the holy syllable, everything comprising Om. Through this tripartite syllable and its fourth, superior dimension, the whole world is connected. Here again we get an insight into the connection between tapas (heat) and Om. Then the renowned Yoga of six is defined as the rule for this (unity): breath restraint (pranayama), senses removal (pratyahara), meditation

(Dhyana), concentration (dharana), contemplation (tarka), absorption (samadhi). This is said to be six times the amount Yoga. MA U 6.18

The possible link between the six-fold yoga of Maitri Upanisad and the eight-fold yoga of Patanjali is speculative. The Eight-fold Way of Patanjali's Yoga consists of control (Yama), exercise (niyama), posture (asana) and restriction of breath (pranayamah), detachment from senses (pratyahara). These are very similar to the Maitri Upanisad. These are very similar. The following results are shown in this six times Yoga: Truly, if the knower removed his mind from the outside and the breathing spirit (prana) put objects of meaning to rest, lead him to remain empty of conceptions afterwards. Since the living person (jiva) who is called the breathing spirit has come from what is not the breathing spirit, therefore, really let the breathing spirit hold the fourth state of his breathing spirit. MA U 6.19

Here, the importance of the prana (respiratory spirit) and its capacity to distract the practitioner from the actual is stressed. When properly used, prana leads to the fourth level of awareness where the Self is understood.

Meditation and correct breathing are the means by which you become aware of samadhi, where this state, Turiya, is felt. The Maitri Upanisad gives more yogic instructions: By taping your tongue to your palate, you see Brahma through meditation in restraining speech, mind and breath. When you see in yourself the bright and subtler Self through suppressing your ego, then when you look at your own self, you become selfless (niratman). MA U 6.20

The path that enables the subtle body to manifest itself from the gross body is another topic that dates back to the Upanisads of Chandogya in the Maitri: the Susumna tube, leads up, transmits the breath, pierces the palate. By entering (yuj) the respiration, Om's syllable and the mind, it is possible to go up. By turning the tip of the lingua against the palate, you can see excellence by connecting the senses together (sam-yojya). Therefore, he's going to egoism. Become a non- experiencer of pleasure and pain by selflessness; he obtains an absolute unity (kevalatva). - After causing the breath that has been restricted to remain standing first, after moving beyond the capped, it can finally have union in the head with the limitless. The union finally would exist in one's head. MA U 6.21

By joining air, mind and the sacred syllable Om, the prana is transferred from the spine base to the head with the correct posture. But in the Principal Upanisads this complex energy movement theory is not further developed. Maitri 6:25 reiterates the meaning of yoga as harmony and peace: whereas one so unites respiration with the syllable Om and the whole multiplicity of worlds. Or maybe you follow them! - Therefore, Yoga (joining) was called (smrta). The unity of breath and mind, and the senses, and the surrender to all living conditions. This is called Yoga. MA U 6.25

The reference to heat follows directly. The warmth here is represented as the fire in his stomach, and is used to burn breaths accompanying sacred syllable Om as a sacrificial fire. Truly as the huntsman draws his net in fish and sacrifices them in the fire of his heart, so definitely do one draw Om in these breaths and give them in the fire free from sickness. It's also liked a caldron fried. Now, when ghee light up in a heated caldron in contact with (hot) grass or wood, definitely the non-breathing hot is called in contact with breaths. MA U 6.26

As for Yoga, the Maitri Upanisad concludes that Brahman is realized if one exercises it successfully for six months: if a person exercises Yoga for 6 months, and is constantly liberated (from the sense), infinite Yoga is perfectly made, supreme and mysterious. MA U. 6.28

Observations

The key Upanisads demonstrate the evolution of yoga and meditation from Vedic rituals of sacrificial flames to internal breathing exercises. Tapas, which means austerity and heat, are the key to this evolution. Nevertheless, Eliade incorporates these seemingly disparate definitions by claiming that heat is produced by rigid practices of ascetics including fasting and standing in the sun. He continues to say that tapas, obtained by fasting, by watching in the presence of flames, etc., are accomplished by holding the breath. In Upanisads, we witness the transition to internal practices that generate heat from external sacrifices. Even though it is only briefly mentioned in the Upanisad Maitri, this heat is used to transfer energy up the body to a channel which connects the subtle energy with the omnipresent Brahman. Later on, this energy has been developed via cakras that are mentioned only briefly in the main roads. Hume says, that in the use of the term Nadi it is evident that the writers of the Upanisads have in mind those same ships which are so thoroughly defined as sources of variously specialized vital energy in the subtle etheric vessel coexisting in the composition of the gross physical body in the human organism in later Hindu texts on yoga and related subjects. The Maitri Upanishad specifically mention the name of Susumna, the main channel so often listed in later texts in relation to the Ida and Pingala sources.

The emphasis on tapas or heat generation continues in West hatha yoga practices today, as described in the introduction. While the religious or spiritual divisions are rarely mentioned in hatha yoga today, there is often a period when the back is warmed up by sun greetings which produce heat by movement and exploitation of the opposites, for example by reaching arms as the feet are grounded or moving hips in one direction and in a torso in the other. Eliade quotes Vyasa, which says that Tapas has the opposites to wear, such as the desire to stand and the desire to sit; The absence of words (kastha Mauna) and acts that could indicate one's thoughts and feelings. There are plenty of interesting research to be done on the development of yogic practices from the time of the key developments to their present state of hatha yoga which exploits the opposites to generate heat. David White argues that in these fires of the yogic austerities (tapas), all visible conflict- between God and man, males and females, etc.- is consumed as it were, as the internalization of the sacrifice. So, we can understand how in the Principal Upanisads the Vedic fire rituals are internalized as the yoga practices of breathing exercises, Om mediation, heat generation and the fourth state of awareness (turiya), which has dissolved the illusion between the person and Atman / Brahman.

Chapter Eight

Yoga in Each of the Four States

Your TRUE SELF does not match your WAKING status with your physical body. Our true Self is all four states behind and beyond. Upon discussing this mystery in detail, Hinduism presents us with a simple understanding structure and a practical method for achieving the Fourth State that provides direct knowledge of an everlasting reality, and transcends the three minimal level of consciousness. In the waking, dreaming, deep sleep and beyond it is important to know all aspects of self and consciousness. To this end, we have outlined the yoga of the following four states; but these overlap largely.

The Power of Consciousness

There is a great power behind the regular movement of consciousness, the shakti of consciousness, which starts this cycle. Nobody can interrupt the waking, dreaming and sleeping cycle every day. We may remain up later but we have to excel in this inner strength.

This Shakti has hidden transformative powers which we can develop. The kundalini Shakti develops into the inner power of consciousness which draws us to the highest consciousness. The movement beyond deep sleep into pure consciousness is based on and is part of the kundaline Shakti's awakening,

Nevertheless, in all teachings on the four States this could not clearly be said. The force of celestial sound is Kundalini Shakti, made up from Sanskrit letters. The strength that arises from the first echo, the Aum, strengthens all of the universe's vibratory powers.

Yoga in the Waking State

Through everything we do, the yoga of awakening seeks to be conscious and aware. This is a philosophy of direct observation through which our universal essence of life is separated from the outer manifestations that are restricted through space and time. Many of us are half asleep for most of the day and are scarcely connected and sustained by our inner perception, thought, imagination, daydreams, habit, enjoyment and lack of self-awareness. True wakefulness is still conscious and experiences the world with indifference, rather than with desire. The universe can't give anything to compare with the depth of life, observation and understanding within us.

In the waking state we all have clear and awakening moments which allow us to take sensible decisions. We all have straightforward moments. But few people are aware of this situation.

It may sound bizarre but we have to stay wake and not fall into mechanical action or compulsive reaction, and become lost in the material world's dream. The central emotions rather than conscious reactions, are basically subconscious. Fear, rage and impulses, unintelligent ways of interacting with the world, is little better than dreams. If we look at our so-called waking state, we find there is little real awakening, but rather distracted or stubborn state of mind.

The waking yoga is an awakening moment by moment. This is endorsed by all of its activities. Many ways of becoming more conscious when you wake up. A yogic goal is to improve these sadhanas and introduce them into others.

Chanting and thinking about Aum is a valuable help for all four states of yoga. When you fall asleep, chant Aum; sing Aum when you wake up in the morning. This helps us to keep waking consciousness all day long and to make it dream and sleep.

To note ourselves as the witness of the waking state— the deeper dimension of our existence with vision, deep sleep and spiritual consciousness— is a crucial practice and not a loss to an outside world but a lack of composition within. The overall development of memory is an improvement.

Taking a chant all day long like Aum Namah Shivaya helps us note our deeper consciousness. However, we have to continually energize the slogan. Simple mechanical replica can lead to a loss of awake consciousness. The most important thing to remember is the Lord every morning by mantra like the hymns of Hinduism, prater smarami.

Brahma Muhurta is the perfect time for meditation, a period of one to two hours before sunrise. It is the moment of the day that you can most easily connect to the divine conscious powers, bring awareness into the waking state behind the deep sleep state and understand how the whole universe is born from Brahman as Aum.

When our mind is drifted into an absence of consciousness, Pranayama brings us back to the deeper energy of consciousness which persists in deep sleep. The more we have such a single prana, the more we can focus our consciousness all day long.

Through using senses for the purpose of meditation instead of amusement or enjoyment, we learn to be mindful of the being's existence and the light of consciousness behind forms of nature. This sadhanas may be further converted into pratyahara or meaning retirement.

This helps us understand the impermanence of all awakening experiences, even traumatic events in our lives.

Karma yoga, selfless service, helps us to sensitize and trigger mechanical reactions in our actions. This is especially important if meditation is difficult. This is vital. Those who continue to be ever awake will never die because they have no origin in their wakening, but in their recognition of the divine presence. To do this we need to be undivided and focused on everything we are doing. This is not possible immediately, but every day we will advance.

Yoga in the Dream State.

We are asleep right now and find a portal in our consciousness that enables us to reach the ever awake state. We must learn to understand this. We must brace ourselves for the sleep moment to transcend our waking selves and their external realities. We can then switch into a meditative state rather than just falling asleep.

It is important to remove all television and technological stimuli at least two hours before you sleep, to be able to move into this state of conscious sleep. Walk a few minutes out into nature, sing or meditate quietly, conduct some rituals with ghee lights or incense. These behaviors erase the annoyed patterns of the day from your mind. When you lie down to sleep, first let the mind go and hold the inner light voluntarily. Remember that you are not body or mind, but your instruments.

To order to regulate the mind in every situation, one must manipulate and train the senses and render the senses aware of an uninterrupted situation of focus. In this scenario, a carrier holds the reins of five horses that are his five senses and clear them strongly and positively to his spiritual objective.

At sunrise, noon and sunset, you can reach this door for clear consciousness illumination. For this reason, the Gayatri mantra targets us not only at the light of the outside sole, but also at the light of the inner sole, the light of consciousness behind the duality of the external world.

With all the different movements of our universe, we wake up and sleep or birth and death. This involves the opening, closing or moving of the eyes, and inhaling and exhaling every breath. Yogis are able to cultivate these transition points, such as gaze fixation or breath-holding. The most important of these is the wake and sleep cycle.

The dream state gives the sensory potential voice, touch, sight, taste and feel to the subtle elements or tanmatitas, imaginative essences behind the sensory potential. In reality, the sensory capacity of the dream state is much greater and better than that of the waking state, but it requires a certain cultivation of the mind and the perception. The dream state allows access to abstract realms of vision, imagination and creativity. These are great realms of imagination, motivation and joy. The cultivation of enhanced sensitivities and creative gestures will enable us to reach the highest dream levels.

Many occultists go on astral journeys— waking and traveling through dreams and the astral world. You understand the dream state's reality. They can be caught by the unconscious ego, delusion and desire, considerable inside dream world, even though they may have different psychic abilities.

There are various meditative approaches that help us to transcend the outside perception of who we are. Many yogis learn to awaken in the subconscious or dream body to enter the hidden realms, without being imprisoned by their delusions. Others are trying to circumvent dream constraints and move directly beyond imagination to formless levels of consciousness. Note that the principal mental fluctuation that Yoga calls for us to master is the imagination in Sanskrit called Vikalpa.

Two elements of dreaming yoga exist. The first is to try and become conscious of the dream state (usually ending our dreams). It doesn't mean being aware of the dream state in our waking self, but rather being aware that we dream, disconnected from body and mind. This enables us to make our dreams more insightful instruments and to realize that dreaming is but a development of our own thought.

The second aspect of this yoga, which is very connected with the bhakti yoga, is to dream of our highest spiritual wishes and longings. It is to foster the higher creative forces, the inventive power of the mind, to reflect a more elevated spiritual reality. Dream is the best way for us to dream our ultimate vision which is to communion with the Lord in divine realms of pure energy, light and joy if we meet the heart and the eternal wishes of our souls. The higher dimensions of Bhakti Yoga

have a peculiar resonance. The vision can become a normal worship state by hearing devotional music, mantra and chanting before sleep. Creative visualization is very useful, especially in the inner visualization of the Divine. Manasa puja is ideal for spiritualizing the dream state. It is a mental puja. When you sleep, remember and share the image of the Deity. You are to worship the Divine in such a way that your heart aspires to your highest hopes in our lives, which are to connect with your greater world through our hearts.

Yoga in Deep Sleep

The yoga of deep sleep mainly holds shapeless consciousness and comes back in the original space or vacuum in which everything has seed shapes. There is no objective reality to observe in deep sleep and no separate self to identify with. World and self-awareness are fused into a state of purity with possibility forces and systems of cosmic concepts or dharma. There are only initial movements, a mass of light, energy and vibration. The body itself is external or form-based. The yoga of deep sleep is conscious of this simple vibration.

By establishing deep sleep consciousness, the higher, formless realms of the causal plane may be reached. These are realms of reflection, vacuity and illumination. Through cultivation of a deeper peace and contentment and through learning to be an unformed, pure mind, without need of an outer world or body, we will gain access to them. We can do this by promoting higher ideals, the concept of universal justice, of peace and harmony. One way to help is to meditate on the yantra or geometric shapes, such as the famous Shri Yantra, of the Deities.

Two levels of yoga from deep sleep. It starts with deep pratyahara or sensory focus and withdrawal in the waking state. Thus, the mind, the pranas and the senses can be drawn into a waking deep sleep state. You keep your consciousness deep inside your brain, and your external mind and senses are closed.

Instead, in the process of deep sleep, you strive to maintain a continuous consciousness, not as a waking identity but as a deeper consciousness behind the eyes. It's the real yoga nidra or sleep.

Another key part of deep sleep yoga is to promote peace and happiness in every day life, particularly the capacity to abandon, relax and acknowledge. During waking condition helps, exercise pratyahara. You have to learn to leave yourself in the undifferentiated state of consciousness of namedness and shape, body and mind. We need to acknowledge the mystery that true know-how transcends the mind and that the mind knows only a dark or unknown shape that at best represents only some sort of light. Deep sleep can then lead us into the state of Turiya.

Yoga Nidra

Yoga nidra is one of mainstream yoga practice's main aspects. Today, its success shows a new interest in ancient practices of yoga. Many forms are now being taught as yoga nidra, but these are only preliminary practices. True yoga nidra is an integral part of four states ' yoga, which wakes, dreams and deep sleeping. In the moment of sleep or rest, it involves moving towards the inner peace of the witness. It allows us to consciously fall asleep as a deep pratyahara and enables us to shut down the motive organs and senses during the awake period as appropriate. We attract our consciousness into the heart in this state, not the physical heart but the deeper spiritual heart. The free stream of knowledge from higher consciousness in the state of yoga nidra, in which one suspends one's mind. This is referred to as the Yoga Sutras as a dharma megha samadhi. We touch the Ishvara consciousness, the inner instructor of yoga, by means of real yoga nidra.

Yoga in the Fourth State

The fundamental activity of awakening, dreaming and profound sleep in the yoga cultivates the consciousness of a witness or Sakshi bhava. Staying strong in the witness state means awakening and sleeping, time and place, birth and death instantly. This concludes with wakeful thought, mindful sleep and consciousness.

Witness cultivation is also the fourth state's main activity, which includes help practices. Firstly, we should maintain a dharmic and mindful lifestyle, as defined in the Yama and Niyama practice of yoga. It involves a vegetarian diet; our sense and motor organs and our mind and emotions being controlled. All this is necessary for any serious practice of meditation. Furthermore, we need to learn to keep awareness moment by moment. It starts with daily morning and evening meditation practices, mantra and certain spiritual qualities, especially astute focus, concentration and uncontaminated observation.

A well-experienced meditator immerses himself, while outer pranas and thoughts float around him. He regulated karmas enough to master the art of no reaction and return to samadhi. With this suitability, he can easily reach in deep sleep the subtle dimensions of the causal plane.

Natural Patterns of Sleep

Sleep because you want to Ensure you have proper operation and wellbeing. In fact, we are scheduled to sleep every night to heal our minds and bodies. The timing of our transitions from wakefulness to sleep is largely determined by two interactors– the internal biological clock and the sleep-wake homeostat. Two interacting devices. These two factors also account for why we usually remain awake during the day and sleep in the night under normal conditions. But what happens exactly when we sleep away? In the early twenties, scientists found sleep to be an inactive brain condition, prior to modern sleep studies. As nightfall and the sensory input from the atmosphere decreased, it was generally accepted that the brain also had a role.

Essentially, scientific experts claimed that during sleep the brain was stopped just to restart once in the morning.

This way of thinking was challenged by an invention in 1929 which allowed scientists to monitor brain activity. Researchers may find that sleep was dynamical and that the brain was very active at times and did not turn off at any time from recordings called electroencephalograms (EEGs). Over time, sleep studies that track eyesight motion and muscle activity using EEG and other instrument indicate two major sleep types. These were characterized by normal electrical patterns in the brain of a sleeping person and the presence or absence of eye movements.

Rapid eye movement (REM) and non rapid eye movement (NREM) rest are the two primary rest types. On an EEG, the sleep of REMs, also referred to as "active sleep," is characterized by low (small) amplitude, strong waves, alpha rhythm and the movements of their eyes. Most dreaming experts agree that these movements of the hand have something to do with dreams. Typically, when you awaken from REM sleep, you say you have dreamed, sometimes amazingly vivid and sometimes strange dreams. In contrast, when awakened from NREM sleep, people report dreaming much less often. Essentially, muscles are temporarily paralyzed during REM sleep in the arms and legs. This is considered a cognitive obstacle to our desires to "act."

NREM sleep may be divided into 3 different phases: N1, N2 and N3. As the stage N1 to N3 progresses, brain waves are slower and coordinated, and their eyes are still intact. The EEGs show high amplitude (large), low-frequency (slow) waves and rolls in Stage 3, the deepest stage of NREM. This process is called sleep "soft" or "slow wave".

Cycling at Night

Sleep usually starts with NREM sleep in healthy adults. The sequence of clearly rhythmic alpha movements coupled with wakefulness leads to N1, the first stage of sleep, characterized by a mixed-frequency, low-voltage pattern. The passage from wakefulness to N1 takes place seconds to minutes after a person nods for the first time. Normally this first N1 period lasts only 1-7 minutes. Next stage is the second stage, N2, which is recorded in EEG recording via sleep spindles and/or K complexes. During N2 sleep, the high voltage, slow-wave behavior of N3, the third stage of NREM sleep, slowly becomes apparent. This is called slow-wave, delta and deep sleep. It usually lasts from 20 to 40 minutes. As the SERM progresses, the brain becomes increasingly difficult to wake a person from sleep and less responsive to external stimuli.

After N3 sleep, there are typically a number of body movements which signals an "ascent" into a lighter stage of NREM sleep. The first REM sleep episode usually precedes a duration of 5 to 10 minutes for N2. Sleep in usually healthy adults covers 20 to 25% of all Sleep.

NREM sleep and REM sleep loop cyclically through the night. In the first part of the night, most NREMs with slow waves occur; episodes of REM sleep, of which one or five minutes may last first, are usually prolonged throughout the night. During a typical night, N3 sleep takes less time than the first in the second cycle and may be missed from subsequent cycles. The average sleep time for first NREM-REM is between 70 and 100 minutes, the average sleep time for second and subsequent cycles is around 90 and 120 minutes. It is unclear why NREM and NEM sleep have a certain alternating pattern throughout the night. Many scientists believe that special cycles of NREM and REM sleep maximize a physical and mental recovery as well as elements of sleep memory consolidation, but this isn't yet confirmed.

This leads to self-examination, which traces the concept to its origins in the heart. You ask "Who am I?" You know. "And his examination examines the inner heart and the inner consciousness profoundly. A study of the essence of the pure" I am "beyond the self of the waking or the physical self. You also investigate the pure" I am "essence that contains our needs and wishes beyond the self of dreams. Eventually, we look beyond the self of deep sleep into the pure" I am, "question the confusion in our lives and understand that our true identity is pure consciousness.

The real self that we discover is not the dreaming self but the dreaming, dreaming and deep sleep of the Self. We usually look for awareness of our wakeful, physical self that is only a dream and an illusion. True spiritual practice starts as we dislodge the waking and waking world, learn to look in and eliminate deeper veils of consciousness.

It is a great help to energize the whole Aum pulse. Bow is Aum, the arrow is our Self-confidence, and as the Mundaka Upanisad states, Brahman or the transcendent state is the aim or objective.

Another form is total surrender to the Lord, known in the Yoga Sutras as Ishvara pranidhana and later as prapatti. This can be followed by a mantra or literally as the highest devotional temperament.

Other People

Just like we normally look at ourselves only according to the waking reality, we do the same with someone, mostly because of their waking reality, when we are engaged actively with them. We should note that every single person and creature, like we do, is subjected to these four states every day. Try to remember that when you look at others you are more than you waking yourself. They are also fused every day into deep sleep and the first reality. We are all in the deep sleep although physically separate. Although we enter the fourth level, Turiya, we become one with all and go beyond body limits and consciousness separations.

Chapter Nine
Dreams & the Astral World

INNER Realms THE INNER INNIVERSE is NOT like the one, but much compatible, complex and logical, and much more advanced than this one we know as a jiva. In this world, Antarloka, there are great schools where students can come together to dream about a more prosperous future when they incarnate. Here they mix and communicate with other souls whose physical bodies sleep and with whom they work and collaborate during the next life cycle. It is both the outer and the inner realms, a well-constructed universe.

The importance of sleep to an adult along the way is that he is able to go further into the lower dream and into the inner schools. The repeated use of mantras, japa yoga after a relaxation by hatha yoga and diaphragmatic respiration, before sleep.

The nominee would have dreamless night when japa is well done and the genuine urge remains to overcome the physical forces of the corpus and enter into the astral learning institutions. There'd be deep sleep. Just before waking up, you may have some seconds to dream, which should be overlooked as the astral body re-enters quickly. But deep sleep without dreaming is an example of the Purusha being completely separated from physical forces and completely untouched and functioning in the Devaloka.

Should dreams be remembered? Are you going to get the tricks? In many cultures, it is almost common to try to remember one's dreams, and even dream scientists interpret for you. All these limits are similar to the domain of superstition and much less attractive than other pragmatic approaches to spiritual growth. A beginner or even one in the medium stage should try to forget his dreams and strengthen the fibers, through frequent sadhanas, of mind and psyche. In reality, after the charya and kriya marga have been well mastered and crossed on the yoga marga, there is a time in which memory of one's songs is positive and fruitful, but only between the guru and the shishya.

It may be helpful if a sat guru leads them every morning, when they arise, to write them down and place them at the end of each month at his heiligen feet. This would strictly be a relationship for guru-shishya training and not more than four months for a specified period. It might be difficult, even disheartening, to make this happen for you. And if you remembered it could take the fact into the awakened world and construct things you don't want to encounter; you'd like to have your dreams when you wake up!

They wish to forget bad dreams as soon as possible, so as not to reinforce them in the immediate subconscious by remembering them in the conscious mind and manifesting them in our everyday lives. It is to build to talk of a bad dream. It must be avoided to forget. Therefore, it is better to let them slip and find them as unimportant and not one part of you if you're least worried about dreams and are not driven by a guru everyday, because you think that a television program is.

Upon performing japa and meditating, a seeker consciously slept. This training has given her access to an indoor school, where her astral body meets others. Upon learning how to join her sat guru in these Second World schools, she avoids dream states that are less energy-efficient.

Chapter Ten

Sleep & Well-Being

It's not just a physical movement but an inner change in consciousness that the evolutionary cycles pass through. It is ultimately linked to the inner forces in eternity which enhance the capability to renovate our body and mind. It does not mean pure physiological energies. The bioclock is the representation of the movement of the Sun outside as we wake in the morning sunlight and sleep after the Sun's setting at night. On the inner plane, the prana and breathing checks our biological clock. We have some 21,600 breaths every day, or one every four seconds, with each and every 24 minutes or 1/60 of the day, according to yogic texts, 360 breaths every.

The subconscious goes along with the respiration and shares the patterns to cycles. The prana, together with the mind, sinks into a withdrawn state during sleep. For another day we reset our biological clock in deep sleep. Obviously, our contemporary activity has brought us from the organic time of nature, determined by mechanical clocks, with our social events. We lived in the night and usually stay up from sunset and fight our biological patterns, starting with the arrival of electricity. Once we recognize our biological rhythms, we are deprived proper sleep and our activities are disturbed physical and psychological.

Our biological clock mandates that one day we live at a time with a new experience each day. Our body, mind and ego are changed every day, but subtle changes take place. We do not have constant time movement, but are modulated or stopped by day and night variations. Every night during deep sleep our consciously returns to an unequivocal state and, almost like a daily life and rebirth, emerges in the morning. Our frequent retreat to subtle realms overshadowed by our fascination with physical existence We underestimate the importance of us. This leads us to assume that our physical identity exists endlessly, which is not the case. Throughout our daily lives, deeper forces of consciousness and creation influence us. So too, one day at a time our spiritual practice gives us new opportunities for growth, transformation and realization of our greater awareness within us and around us every day. Our spiritual life benefits from learning to take on the unique power and transformation of every day.

Mind & Prana

In the four states, our mind and prana radically change. The mind and prana are actively engaged in the wakeful state. The mind is trapped in dualistic waves, like and hate, pleasure and pain, love and hatred, with desire and repulsion. The prana is enveloped by two alternating currents of breathing and exhalation, sensation and motion and energy changes on the left and right sides of the body. The mind is pulled inwardly in a dream state and our prana turns inward. Our inner mind is enlightened and allows us to radically change the perceptions in time and space. We also undergo a more subtle non-physical prana, which projects a shifting dream body based on mind thought. We operate effectively in the astral body, comprising of pranamaya, manomaya and vijnanamaya koshas, as we dream. The dreams of pranamaya are mostly energy-intensive in nature. Sensory and emotional are Manomaya dreams. Dreams of Vijnanamaya correspond with more personal perspective to meditations of the deep sleep.

The subconscious is merged with a state of delay in deep sleep. Prana supports the body, supporting it from its seed state. We have a deep natural pratyahara, sensual abstinence in which all our faculties return to their core energies. (This is discussed at length in Prashna Upanishad) In the fourth state, prana and mind are merged into a more profound consciousness for those who are able to experience this through meditation. The mind stops making its own gestures, acts only as a unitary consciousness device, and is no longer capable of producing false ego behaviors. We must abandon our affiliation with the body to enter the fourth cycle and remove the Prana knot the binds us to it. It is said that our consciousness resides in the eyes in the waking state, especially in the right eye. This dwells in the throat in the dream state. It resides in deep sleep— the heart, not physical or emotional organ, is the deeper spiritual center. It is also concentrated in the organ of the fourth state, but not consciously, as in deep sleep.

Healing

The root of all deeper healing is to draw our prana, or precious energy within us. The prana of deep sleep has the unique power to heal all the other pranas and the mind in this way. The brain may take away negative habits and resources and restart its equilibrium in deep sleep. In all psychological healing this is important. However, the greatest heal of the body is also attributed to a deep sleep consciousness and prana. A yogi may access and direct this inner power of prana by his hands or eyes to both guide and heal his disciples.

Sleep and the Home

Most of us describe our homes as sleeping, indicating the value of sleep. The most private room in the house is our bedroom. All of us expect to go home and have a good night's rest, particularly after a busy day or some time away. It's a huge pain to have no home or place to sleep. The cornerstone of our sense of well-being is to build our home or place of rest. Sleeping in the same place gives us some inner comfort.

Nonetheless, it's not just a matter of a house, a room or a physical home. Sleep brings us again in our sacred home, in which deep sleep renews us. Divine strength and awareness. This positive effect is felt by us all. If we have life challenges, we all want to go back to the rest of our houses, where we can shut down, relax, get away, and sleep well. We are all happy to be asleep as we know that rest leads to a normal state of peace and well-being where the responsibility of the planet can be published. Sleep is the same for either beggar or king. This tranquility of deep sleep will help us understand our deeper consciousness ' calm. It is not necessary to rest in our outdoor home, however. We have to learn to relax in our internal house.

Chapter Eleven
Science & the Mind

India's Culture has made inner consciousness into its primary concern over the past several years.

Dharmic culture considers the most important ways of awareness and the most basic endeavor of lives are inquiries into the nature of consciousness. This inner understanding is the greatest science, as it alone allows us to really understand the nature of the universe, its creation and its meaning, and also the existence of our inner being, one with all.

Modern science gradually develops a new understanding of consciously through its many new research ventures better aligned with progressive dharma than with the old, set, physical vision of the world. This comes in two directions of awareness.

In order to clarify the coherency of natural laws, quantum physics provides, first, a unitary field of consciousness behind the cosmos. This universal field of perception is only a theory so far. But the pure consciousness behind the world, the Vedic concept of God, the Divine, or the Supreme Truth is well-known in Vedic thought as Brahman, and the origin and finality of all.

The second pragmatic approach to consciousness is modern psychology, including brain mapping, functions and forces, and the practice of how these affect the mind and awareness, like sleep and dreams. A latest method of brain research shows the healing power of yoga, mental health therapy and the workings of neurology.

Nevertheless, modern science is far from recognizing the Absolute Reality of consciousness. The problem is that Neuroscience describes the brain as the center of thought, consciousness and physical reality. In this context, the main method of treating mental dysfunctions remains chemical medicine.

Hindu philosophy teaches us that brain, mind and consciousness are related, but in reality, they are different. The physical brain is a device for the mind, but the mind has an abstract dimension that extends through physical reality. The core mind, our karmic patterns, places our body at death and brings us to another body and life– many yogis are very well aware of mystics and occultists.

However, neither is the mind, which has its own structure, works and is part of nature. Such a Presence over body and mind is an instrument for deeper consciousness, the true Self, the real source of consciousness and beyond all transformation, motion, time and space. The atman is the supreme consciousness of Brahman. Human perception is inseparably connected to the embodied consciousness or mind.

The symbolic brain of energy and consciousness, the thousand-petallic lotus, the highest of the 7 chakra yogical thought, is metaphorically placed behind the physical brain and its chemistry. This houses the keys of higher consciousness, but must be triggered by yogic practices. In the ordinary person it's mostly latent or uncharted.

If modern science tests the brain for consciousness, it is like testing a man by looking at his shadow's movements. Hindu thinking tells us how to first transcend the mind and its biological limitations and compulsions and then how to transcend the individualized mind to go beyond our karmic boundaries. It ultimately leads us to find pure information, a simple concept all widespread. It takes us to the core of our consciousness that continues to wake, dream and sleep.

Section I

1. Aum. The unpalatable Aum syllable is all. His explanation now follows. It's only Aum, what was and what is and will be. And that is also all Aum, after these three periods of time. It's all Brahman. That. Brahman is the Self (atman). This Self is four-four.

2. Section II

3. The disappointer of what is gross, that is Vaishvanara, the universal individual, the first quarter of Aum, dwells in the waking state, with outside awareness, with seven limbs and nineteen mouths.

4. The enjoyer of what is subtle, that is Taijasa, luminous, the second quarter of Aum is living in a dream, with an inner awareness of seven limbs and nineteen mouths.

5. You don't have any wishes or dreams when you sleep, Sushupti. In the deep sleep state, one's awareness, a mass of knowledge, is brought together. This is the state of happiness, with the joyfulness of the single mouth. Prajna is the third quarter of Aum, the power of wisdom.

6. This deeply sleeping state is the master of all, the master of everything, the interior controller, the foundation of all, the origin and the end.

7. Where there is no inward awareness; no external knowledge; no mixed inner or outer knowledge; in which there is no mass of knowledge; where there is no knowledge, where there is no absence of knowledge; where there is an intangible, beyond all signs, without meaning, evident, that is, the which is the substance of the experience, beyond the real, metaphysical and non binary universe, of the unitary self. This is Self. This is Self. We know that That.

Section III

1. You should know this Self as the unperishable Aum, quarter and scales, by the letters A- Kara, U-Kara, M-Kara—the letters A, U and M.

2. The waking condition and Vaisvanara are the first test of letter A, the first fourth. It penetrates everybody as its heart. You fulfill all desires and you know that first and foremost.

3. The dream state and Taijasa is the second variable, the letter U. Big, one gets a consistency of awareness, equanimity and keeping both other states, dream and deep sleep. There is no foreign Brahman who knows this in his home.

4. The deep sleep condition and Prajna, the third step in the letter M, is the indicator of the dissolution of all things. The entire universe that knows this is weighed and dissolved.

5. The fourth state, Turiya, which does not include knowledge, the termination, auspicious and non-dual, of the amazing universe, Aum; that's the Self. He joins into the Self by himself.

Commentary

Aum is the whole universe, all time and all eternity. This Aum is our essential nature in the 4 waking, dreaming, profound sleep and the four quarters of Turiya. All the time comes from it, beginning with our life's movement. This is the four aspects of our nature; which Agni symbolizes as a fire of life and consciousness.

Vaishvanara is the root energy of the waking state, the human soul in a waking condition, for digestive capacity. The 7 limbs are the 7 secret prana energies. The nineteen mouths are the five sensory organs, the five motor organs, the five tanmatras, the four facets of mind (Aahamkara, ego, manas, spirit, buddhi, intellect and chita, sub-conscious spirit and memory).

The dreaming state often includes ruminations in the subconscious mind, revives historic events, exposes good times and anxieties regarding things that disrupt the mind. Here a man dreams of happy moments with his mother, the summer day, when he and a friend find a mango tree with mature fruit.

The fire of the mind is Taijasa. It represents memory and the implicit essence of our awakening experience, which connects us to the abstract worlds as well. This implicit body has the same form and strength as the physical body but consists not of matter but of energy.

In the heart of our dreams, Prajna is the inner fire of wisdom. All happiness in life is due to our ability to reach the bliss or Ananda, which is transmitted to us through deep sleep rest.

The true Self is not an external entity known by the mind. It is an unmistakable witness to all events. It goes beyond three stages, waking, dreaming and sleeping and is known only by going beyond these three stages and their energies.

The four states reflect the four facets of Aum as A, U, M and afterwards silence. Aum is the universal consciousness pulse, the Self's very echo. The first state of awakens is and retains our consciousness ' principal experience. The dream state experiences both deep and wakeful sleep, all of which form part of a larger vision. Everything is consumed by deep sleep. The transcendent fourth, the state of absolute harmony, lies behind these fluctuating conditions. You should know that in all of them is the same Self and fire of consciousness.

Chapter Twelve

The Great Cosmic Dream

Our life is only a long sleep and a vision, not of a pure personal existence but of our spirit, who has had many lives in various bodies. Our bodily lives depend upon the forgetfulness of our eternal roots and the appeal of a temporary external reality, where we lose our true spiritual identity and become the physical body. How long does our physical life go? As long as a lifetime, most of us will respond. The reality is that the lack of sleep kills our physical consciousness every day. We spend about 8 hours a day in sleep or about a third of our lives. We are much less conscious of the sleep than we are of the waking state. We do not take sleep seriously or consider it as real except as a waking state epiphenomenon. But there are many secrets in the waking state, including the key,

The Fact of Impermanence

The most distinctive thing in a dream is that it is just a momentary affair with no lasting result or continuity in the outside world. In the waking state, you can't visit your dream places. After a dream has ended, it's forgotten fast. We can have great success or great difficulty in dreaming but we don't generally take it seriously when we awaken.

While the waking state is lasting more than dreaming, there are similar time constraints. It also ceases finally and has to be forgotten. The wakeful state is a kind of lengthy collective dream. We enter a state of wakefulness which is fixed in nature, which we call the material world. But if you look deep, you'll see every second of the physical reality. Modern physics has dissected physical reality and has shown that in the vast advanced society of space and light it is an illusion of small particles and energy fields. The material world's apparent stability reveals its illusionary reality through ongoing changes.

The movement of the day is transitory, with morning and night quickly changing. An hour can pass so quickly that we don't know it. The transition from season to year is a major factor in the development and enhancement of the natural world. During the spring the outward rush of prana accompanies in the autumn the internal retreat. Our own ageing by our biological clock is most significant and shows that our physical body is not a permanent phenomenon but a time-limited movement. And even in a few minutes or hours of time, our mind changes more quickly than the body.

The length of our lives reflects the meaning of our dreams. In the end– although it may seem like things last, however much we win or lose– they end up being nothing, whether yesterday's food, our own children's experiences or our adult lives ' achievements. The pain of those people who die young reflects the unforeseen transience of life. None of us can really be sure that this is our last day.! This reality is profoundly felt by most of us, for example, in older family homes, and find that they have changed radically or are no longer. During the course of time, we all lose our friends and family. Often, especially when we get older, the world loses interest in us. Even if big world leaders die, they too will be forgotten in a few weeks ' time. The time is constant and does not leave anything at all.

The experience of impermanence forms the foundation for great art and literature, particularly tragic events. We're so sad that we're really going to die ourselves. But we can not see the profound truth of our life, which is not bound to time, in our search for the eternal existence. We must be beyond the illusion of time created by our daily cycles of waking, dreaming and deep sleep in order to discover that immortal soul. We forget our cosmic truth and become a small, outward- looking consciousness in the ignorance of deeper sleep. The ego's stupor leads us to accept our physical body as our true nature and to forget about the origins of consciousness within us. We are left with deep sleep's mysterious capacity by waking and dreaming.

The Illusion of the Senses

The physical universe is a representation of the physical senses, or phantasmagoria. Our sense about sight gives us our main world image or definition. Sound interacts with us. More physical stimuli are created by touch, taste and smell. Nevertheless, the senses do not give a sense of what is true. Sensory images are evocative and quickly activate our imagination, which is a dreamlike characteristic that creates visions of what we want to do or what our senses bring to us. For instance, a beautiful woman has different effects on the men's senses from the women. A hungry man's smell of food is better than a man who's just eaten it. Biological imperatives are triggered by our senses and we have to act.

We spend a great deal of time assessing our chosen truth, regardless of whether it's what we are really buying or relationships. Intelligence needs to be developed in order to distinguish between what is and what is not. Vedic philosophy teaches us that the entire world is but a snapshot, like reflections from a depth of consciousness in a mirror. In truth, the sensory perception is a vision as much as it is a seeing or an awareness. Our senses are so much the ability to imagine and wish as a tool for assessing objectively the essence of any concrete reality.

We know the famous tale of five blind men how, thanks to their limited contact, everyone comes to a different conclusion about the existence of an elephant. Our five senses remind us of the world that can distort or confuse us as much as clarity. It is necessary to see who we really perceive behind the five senses and the ephemeral physical organ. Most people live more in imagination than in simple awakening consciousness in the current era of information technology. We've invested in virtual reality, photos of social media and digital profiles that aim to represent us. It is in fact easy to see whether we simply analyze our conscientious behaviors all day long and how much we want and visualize our physical reality.

Each Life Is a Day in the Lifetime of Our Soul.

The daily step from waking to dreaming and deep sleep represents our souls ' duration of travel from one person's life to another. Waking concerns our stay in physical reality, the universe of dense matter and form. In yogic philosophy, this involves the universe. Dream is the world of subtle form, thought and energy that we live in celestial reality. Sometimes this is called the moon's atmospheric domain in yogic thought. Deep sleep refers to our stay in the shapeless, causal realms of light and seed energy. In yogic teachings (Prashna Upanishad) this involves the sky, the atmosphere or the sun.

Sleep, dream and everyday reawakening mimic the experience of death and rebirth. Death is only a sleep in which we dream uncannily and wake up in a new physical form. We are, as it were, born and died every day. In the morning, the self that wakes up is somewhat different from the self that was sleeping the evening before. Every night we leave something and every morning we take something new. Most people forget about this everyday change in nature, but it's easy for those who know that. Try to think before you go to bed in the night, and consider this when you wake up in the morning. What it was isn't unusual to forget. Making our day-to-day sleep shift allows us to master the greater path of our soul through the physical, astral and causal realms. We will conquer death and transcend all space and time when we can live fully in consciousness one day. Day and night mysteries are strong.

Every Day as the Creation of the Entire Universe

Deep sleep is associated with Mula Prakriti, the universe's root material. We will reach into the middle of life if we can stay conscious and study it. Every day, through the divine Aum vibration, we will witness the development from pure consciousness to great materiality. The consciousness, the creator, sustaining and transforming Ishvara of all that our soul is one, lies behind deep sleep. Why Ishvara allows and absorbs everything can be felt every day. This Ishvara is the Adi Guru or initial yoga instructor, as is taught in the Yoga Sutras, by the cosmic vibration Aum. This divine creative process is represented by our human minds.

But, at all times, all life is present. The passage of time as Brahma every day and night represent the withdrawal of the world, as the universal creation is the day and the night. Eternity is the never- ending day of pure consciousness whose dual shadows form our external world of reality, day and night. This is our daily experience before we remove ignorance from our minds.

Likewise, each sphere point is the Infinite, overflowing with many brahmandas, or universal eggs, which evolve different world systems.

Chapter Thirteen

Conclusion

Learn how to turn your everyday activity into a consciousness regular adventure. Observe with intense attention the shifts of waking, dreaming and sleep as they include many secret doors to higher awareness. Cultivate a consciousness moment by moment to always be alert. Note, each day as a stage in its celestial unfoldment, your endless wandering of consciousness. Know your regular movements from dream to sleep and learn how they influence your body, mind and prana. Wake up in your ever-waking Self. Note that falling asleep or losing consciousness is a significant calamity. Every day as the last day, the Everlasting Life's everlasting day. Try every day to discover your everlasting ability. Adapt to the power of awareness which moves you through the three states. Allow it to take you over. The inner directing of the drama and fate of your life is your consciousness. Turiya is not a State other than the bigger states, but as super consciousness penetrates all layers of reality. Ramana Maharishi considers Turiya to be the only truth as the natural state which permeates the other Ones. The Mandukya Upanishad talks of Turiya as a pure consciousness that the mind cannot explain, cannot understand and cannot be understood, but eventually realized as the one true self. Because of its unique nature, Turiya cannot be represented by any empirical science instrument. It has no unique or generic features, it's one without a second

www.ingramcontent.com/pod-product-compliance
Lightning Source LLC
Chambersburg PA
CBHW051028030426
42336CB00015B/2775